THE *Real* SKINNY ON WEIGHT LOSS SURGERY

*An Indispensable Guide
to What You Can REALLY Expect!*

Written For Real People, By Real People!!

Julie M. Janeway
Karen J. Sparks
Randal S. Baker, M.D., F.A.C.S.
with
Carrie A. Liebrock, R.D.
Scott H. Glass, M.S., M.A., L.L.P.

Foreword by

Judith Brown Clarke
Olympic Medalist, World Record Holder
Sports Illustrated® Sportswoman of the Year

Illustrations by
Liz Rehfuss

Little Victories Press

THE *Real* SKINNY ON WEIGHT LOSS SURGERY

An *Indispensable* Guide to What You Can REALLY Expect!

ISBN Print Ed. (10 digit) 0-9767672-8-7 (13 digit) 978-0-9767672-8-2
Library of Congress Control Number 2005924894

Cover Design:
Robert Aulicino, Pro Art Graphics
www.aulicinodesign.com

Illustrations & Graphics:
Liz Rehfuss
Lansing, Michigan

Printer:
Data Reproductions, Inc.
Auburn Hills, Michigan
www.datareproductions.com

Book Layout & Interior Design:
Suzette Perry, Infinity Graphics
Okemos, Michigan
www.infinitygraphics.com

Authors' Promotional Photos:
Tom Nakielski, Lights On Studio
Lansing, Michigan
www.lightsonstudio.com
and
Robert Neumann, Big Event Studios
Grand Rapids, Michigan
www.bigeventstudios.com

Promotional Graphic Design:
Liz Rehfuss
Lansing, Michigan
www.angelwingimages.com

Copyediting:
Lorna Lane
Lansing, Michigan
and
Sally Cannon, Ph.D.
Bay Harbor, Michigan
and
Eugenie "Coco" Cook
Jackson, Michigan

Promotional Photo Hair and
Make-up Design:
Saul Rodrigues & Danielle Ruehle
Steven L. Marvin Salon
and Wellness Spa
(An Aveda® Salon)
East Lansing, Michigan
www.stevenlmarvin.com

Web site Design:
Wojo Design, LLP
Freeland, Michigan
www.wojodesign.com

Published by:
Little Victories Press
4371 Kinneville Road, Suite 200
Onondaga, MI 49264

www.LittleVictoriesPress.com

— DEDICATION —

This book is dedicated to all those REAL people out there who are tired of dealing with their serious weight issues, and want to improve their health and quality of life. This book is for every person who has battled the scale and lost, missed far too many experiences and opportunities because of their weight, and for those whose precious lives are being shortened every minute because of health problems associated with their weight. This book is for all of you who are overweight and afraid.

For you, we offer a look at an alternative. It's not a cure, and it's not for everyone. We offer you the opportunity to investigate, to learn, and to see what real people who've had weight loss surgery go through. We offer you a choice, and maybe a chance at better health and a better life. At the very least we offer you information, and hope that there is something out there that will help you help yourself.

If you are choosing to read this book, we applaud you for your courage in continuing the fight to live life on your own terms. You deserve to get the most out of every minute life has to offer. You deserve to make the choices concerning what you do and don't experience, not have them made for you based on your size and weight. You are beautiful, you are not alone, and you are worth whatever it takes to be happy and healthy in your own body. It is for you, all our kindred spirits in the world, that we dedicate this labor of love.

━ A C K N O W L E D E M E N T S ━

On behalf of Little Victories Press, Karen and I would like to extend our tremendous gratitude to the following people and businesses for their amazing support, assistance, trust, and belief in LVP and this project. Without you this book would not have come into existence, and the entire "REAL Skinny" series of books regarding weight loss surgery would not have been conceived. You are all permanently part of the Little Victories family, and to each of us personally, you will always be family as well: Dr. Randal Baker who made all this possible, the staff at MMPC® CFHE, who helped Dr. B., Judi Brown Clarke who is such a wonderful person and tremendous grounding force, Carrie Liebrock who reminds us to love animals and love ourselves, Scott Glass, who reminds us that with faith all things are possible, Dawn Baker for reading until she was blind, being patient, supportive and kind, and Dr. Baker's family who gave up so much time with him to allow him to be such an integral part of this endeavor, Robert Aulicino who did such a tremendous job on the cover design, and our dear friends Eugenie "Coco" Cook and Judy Burgess who never doubted for a second.

We never would have finished without the help of Kim Colton from Data Reproductions (you're a goddess), the staff at Data Reproductions (best printers on the planet), and Suzette and Brian Perry at Infinity Graphics, and Liz Rehfuss (world's best "save the day" graphic artists). We'd also like to thank Jerry and Clarice Baker, Wojo Design, Tom Nakielski of Lights On Studio, Robert Neumann, Steven L. Marvin, Saul Rodrigues, Danielle Ruehle, Dr. Sally Cannon, Dr. Louis Cannon, Sue and Charlie Hilton, Theresa Martone, Kimberly Stump, Gail Sobecki, Tonnie Drake, Brad Sweda, Barb Ford, Karen Kay, Dave Westcot, and all the men who participated in the research for Chapter Ten. You have all been great, and we thank you for the contributions each of you made individually to this undertaking.

We would each like to make some personal acknowledgements as well.

JULIE

Mine will be the longest as I have a tremendous number of people to thank. Without most of them I wouldn't even be alive to write this book. I love you all. First I'd like to thank my husband Matt who amazingly didn't kick me to the curb during this grueling process. Thanks for your support, belief in me, and for loving me fat, loving me thinner, and loving me at all. Secondly, to my mom who never waivered in her belief in me, this surgery, or this book: thanks for taking care of me, and for your proofreading and copyediting. Great job mom. To my sister Cheryl for her wise words. Thanks for the motivation. Luv ya. To my dad: thanks for really getting behind this one dad, and thanks for all those long nights in the hospital. To my niece Meggie: thanks for being such a loving little kid, and for inventing funny words. To my niece Haleigh and my nephew Devin: you guys are awesome and I am so grateful for your love and belief in me. To my brother-in-law Darius: thanks for not shooting me down on this one. I appreciate that very much.

I would especially like to thank the following people because they took a mangled, barely alive woman and put her back together. You have indeed rebuilt me: better, stronger, faster. I am the 6 million dollar woman, and now I'm using my abilities to make the world a better place! Lifelong gratitude goes out to: Dr. John Stubbart, Dr.

John Iaccobucci, Dr. Margie White, Mickey Loomis, Dr. Edmond Ducommun, Craig Mefford, Dr. Edward Cook, Dr. Ann Hakkila, Dr. Randal Palmitier, Dr. Roy Meland, Dr. Charles Bill, Dr. Doug Leppink, Tammy Westfall, Sister Gates, the therapists and staff at Sparrow Rehabilitation, the nurses and medical staff at Spectrum Hospital, and everyone else who helped put Humpty Dumpty back together again! And last, but never least, I would like to thank the good Lord for keeping me on this planet, for giving me what I needed when I needed it, and for bringing me out of the dark to see what I was meant to do.

To Karen: Well, you know… and I know you get it. "Nuff said. Get some sleep.

KAREN

Where to begin….

It is difficult at best to express in words the feelings of gratitude and love to those who most influence your life. I have known since I was a very little girl that my station in this life was to assist others in their journey. Some individuals I have known for many years and others I met for only a moment in time to somehow impact their life. Friends and family alike, to all these individuals I owe thanks as the impact they made on my life has helped to shape me into the person I am today, and provided me with what I needed to write this book.

To my parents, Everett and Barbara Sparks, who have always told me no matter what I was pursuing, (and they will tell you I have pursued many things) "you can do anything you set your mind to." I love you so very much. Thank you for your love and unwavering support in my need to do the "next" thing. And despite my current successes, you know there will always still be something "new" for me to learn and do.

To Julie, there are people you meet in your life who become friends and acquaintances and they enter and exit as time passes for whatever reason. Then there are those special people God puts in your life who just "know you." I believe God saved and healed you from your accident to save and heal me. Thank you for just being you. We did it my friend, we actually did it. Now…I wish you only "good" dreams…go to sleep, we have so very much more to do. God's not done with us yet.

DR. BAKER

I would first of all like to thank my wife Dawn for supporting me through the writing of this book, and life in general. A special thanks to Courtney, Arielle, Jordan, Olivia, Seth, Tessa, Caleb, Isaac, and Titus for allowing their dad to have some time to write and review chapters, even while on vacation!

I would also like to acknowledge Julie and Karen for having the vision and gumption to see this book through to completion. I have never seen any two people work so hard in such an organized way to get the facts about obesity and obesity surgery out to the lay public. Their zeal is truly motivational.

I would like to thank my partners Drs. James Foote and Paul Kemmeter for their support and esteemed character. It is a rare thing indeed to have such highly competent and truly caring surgeons as partners. Thanks also go out to our entire office staff who work tirelessly and care deeply about the welfare of the patients with whom they come in contact. Keep up the good work!

Finally, I would like to thank the Lord for His grace and for giving me such an awesome wife and family, and for allowing me to work with such wonderful people!

TABLE OF CONTENTS

— FOREWORD —

Judith Brown Clarke

I have always believed that "everything happens for a reason." Everything happens in order to teach us some lesson, and to give us some message about what our next step in life should be. Unfortunately, it is often quite a challenge to figure out the nature of that message. I also believe there are other instances, however, when the timing of the lesson is gauged by our ability to handle, or openness to recognizing and accepting the message. This may just be one of those instances. I believe you've picked up this book, written by these particular people, at this time in your life, because you are ready for the lesson, and ready to really hear the message.

And what is the lesson? The lesson is to read this information, examine your life, ask the hard questions, and find a way to do for yourself what you need to do. And what is the message? The message is *live! Live life like the gift that it is. Live it fully, completely, and happily. Live it as a competitor in the game, and not just an observer in the stands.*

Getting back in the game of life is exactly what this book is designed to help you do; surgery, or no surgery. This book will hopefully cause you to think about many aspects of your life. Do you want to continue to cheer only for others, or would you really like to feel the freedom of the run and the roar of the crowd, knowing it's all for you?

It's very easy for any of us to become an observer rather than getting out there in the race and chasing the dream. Life's tough and full of many hurdles, but do you want to know you've overcome them, or would you rather watch the whole race run by you, and find yourself left sitting in the bleachers when the race is done and the people have all gone home?

It's kind of like watching a soap opera and vicariously living through the characters on the screen. What kind of life is that? (By the way, have you noticed that they never listen to you as you shout out valuable information that would save them from six weeks of bad story line?) I understand wanting to sit down and give up when the race gets hard, but the most important thing is being in the race, and not just watching it go by.

As a former Olympian (and yes, I *really* miss my former body), I understand what it means to set goals, make sacrifices, and train hard. I understand the victories and the losses. I understand the effort required to overcome the hurdles. (No, I really mean I understand it. I ran the 400-meter hurdles!) But, the most important and valuable lessons I have learned are from just being in the "game." It is not important whether you win or lose ... okay sometimes it is ... but in general, just being a participant has taught me more about myself than any medal or trophy I have won. Those were the lessons, and because of them I have internalized the message and truly lived.

I can hear what you're thinking now: "If you were a world-class athlete in great shape, how can you know what I feel? How can you know what it's like to be overweight and living with so many restrictions and limitations?" Well, in some ways I do, and you're right, in some ways I don't.

Many people think that athletes can't relate to people with weight problems. In fact, all my life I've carried more weight than I should. When the game you're in measures probable success or failure based on percentage of body fat compared to other competitors, and you're found to be in an "unacceptable range," you come to identify on a certain level with people who have weight issues. Your self-esteem, and self-confidence take a bit of a beating, and in that respect, it's relative.

Now, I don't profess to have experienced the prejudice, the physical pain, or even much of the emotional pain many of you have experienced. But, I can tell you that even if you are in an "unacceptable range" of body fat, you can still show the world that you can not only play the game at a world-class level, but you can win. I did, and you will too.

The reason I know you can play this game and win is because it has nothing to do with physical ability, talent, or skill. It has to do with belief in yourself, and belief in those you choose to help you. You have to work at it, believe it will happen, and make it happen. That's all it takes to reach a goal.

Athletes have to train and work at reaching their goal every day, just like weight loss patients. We're just two ends of the same spectrum – each trying to craft the body into something it's not, and yet something it needs to be. For athletes, sometimes it takes longer than expected to reach a desired level, or an injury slows them down. In either case they just have to work through the frustration, the disappointment, the waiting, and stay committed. They have to rely on the direction of their coaches, hear the cheer of their supporters, keep their eyes on the goal, and rely on their own inner strength.

When you're struggling to lose weight, it takes a long time to reach a desired level, sometimes longer than expected. Instead of injuries, you deal with related medical conditions that delay you and slow you down. But just like athletes, you have to work through the frustration, the disappointment, the waiting, and stay committed. You must rely on the direction of your multi-disciplinary medical team, hear the cheer of your supporters, and most importantly you must keep your eye on the goal, and rely on your own inner strength.

Perhaps each of the challenges or barriers we face in life is actually strength training for the soul. When you're physically strong, it's amazing how much easier external challenges can be, but the same holds true for internal strength. When you rely on your inner strength, it's amazing how much easier personal challenges can be; how much easier it can be to move beyond the lack of validation, or self-imposed barriers. We all have physical barriers of some kind that can hold us back from where we want to be, barriers to move beyond.

As far as external barriers go, it always strikes me how strongly I react to the word "no." If you tell me I can't, then it's the first thing I'll do. I'll do it just to prove to you I can, and to prove you wrong. I'll find the inner will to move that boundary you placed around me out of the way. I decide what my boundaries are, not anyone else.

Now, don't get me wrong, I have a healthy respect for boundaries. Sometimes boundaries keep us from flying off in all directions. When boundaries aren't meant for structure, however, and they're only there to inhibit, that's when the problems start. The worst of these boundaries, of course, are the ones we impose on ourselves.

We lead ourselves to believe that those boundaries cannot be moved except by a miracle. I believe, however, that you can create miracles if you really set your mind to it. Remember: when something positive happens that is not anticipated, that's a miracle. Not all miracles are of biblical proportions. Sometimes they're just little, unexpected victories that let you know you're on the right track.

When you commit yourself to achieving a goal that moves what previously seemed immovable, that is the foundation of a miracle. If you stay committed, find the right help, stay strong, and never stop believing, watch for the miracle to happen. You have everything you need to create your own miracle, and this book is hopefully going to help you start down the road toward it, in whatever direction it may lay.

The direction you'll take after reading this book will only be determined by you, but your guides along the way are some pretty incredible people who've walked a mile in your shoes, or helped others who've walked in your shoes. (You know what they say: you have to walk a mile in another man's shoes … because then you'll be a mile away and have his shoes!) Julie Janeway and Karen Sparks have walked your path, and they know your struggles. They are your kindred souls.

I have always prided myself on my ability to identify people with true souls. This ability is not unlike the way alien abductees explain how they just "know" other alien abductees; they just feel a strange connection. Of course alien abductees then look for the "probe" mark on the back of the other person's neck to confirm their suspicions, but I haven't quite found any such external marking that confirms the true souls I meet.

When I met Julie six years ago in the first of many laborious doctoral classes, I felt a strange connection to her. I immediately heard her soul, and our friendship was born. Now granted, I did see a probe mark on the back of her neck … but that's another story....

Throughout my friendship with Julie, she has struggled with her weight. She has swung on the "rationale" pendulum from "God made me this way, therefore I should be grateful," all the way across to the self-loathing "I am fat, therefore I eat. I eat, therefore I am fat." But to the world, Julie was always just Julie. Her attitude was, "Here I am world, and what are you going to do about it?!" Inner turmoil safely hidden away, Julie has always compensated for lost self-esteem with her tremendous intellect, and an incredible sense of humor.

Julie's sense of humor has carried her through a lot of tough times in her life. I'm sure many of you reading this book can relate. Throughout Julie's struggle with her weight, and the life-altering journey that started with her miraculous comeback from a death-defying car accident, and took her through gastric bypass surgery, she has never lost her ability to laugh. We all need to laugh. Julie, Karen, and the others will help you laugh because life's too short not to.

I've always thought that my ability to find humor in *everything* was a character flaw. I've since come to discover, however, that it is the foundation of strength, and the essence of a quality life. The ability to laugh, to "let go," and to move forward is truly a gift we should cherish. The authors are sharing this gift with you in abundance in this book. Through all of the tough times I watched Julie fight through in the last four years, she's shown incredible strength, courage, and laughed her way to regaining her competitive status in the game of life.

Not only did Julie get back in the game, she dragged Karen back into the game while she was at it. When Julie introduced me to Karen, I thought: "It is true … birds of a feather do flock together." Julie and Karen are like peas in a pod. On the day I first met Karen, the introduction part was quite short, because there really was no need for small talk. We just quickly moved into the comfort of a new friendship. It was like unhooking your bra at the end of the day: a welcome relief.

This comfortable feeling of being with good friends is one of the best features of this book. Throughout it you will feel as though you are part of a personal conversation with Julie and Karen, as well as with Dr. Baker, Carrie, and Scott. That is what I liked most about the book's tone, the ability to address a sensitive subject in a real-life, non-threatening, person-to-person manner.

The clear-cut, informative, "here-it-is, do-with-it-what-you-will" style of this book, is refreshing and honest. You'll find very funny parts mixed with very serious and engaging parts – sort of like real life. But most importantly, what you'll find is the motivation and knowledge to make a decision whether you want to work toward getting back in the game, or pack a picnic and stay in the stands.

As an athlete, and a person who has immense respect for the human body, I jumped at the chance to write the Foreword of this book because I believe in any medically sound method for becoming healthier and increasing life participation. It matters not to me whether you choose to have weight loss surgery. If you simply find the will to try and reclaim control of your health, then I applaud your strength and your Olympian efforts to save your own life.

My background has instilled in me admiration for strength, commitment, and tenacity. I've competed against the world's top track athletes, and even if I lost, I respected the work that went into their performance. For those of you who are struggling with your weight, I understand your struggle, and I admire the fortitude, commitment, and tenacity you are showing in simply reading this book. You are the real winners – the real champions. You are the everyday people who deserve the medals for perseverance and determination. When you choose not to give up, when you choose life, you are American heroes.

If you choose to have weight loss surgery, know that the information you are receiving in this book is accurate, reliable, and necessary for the creation of your game plan. Know that it's okay if you choose surgery, and okay if you don't. Neither is a cop out. As long as you've really investigated the options, learned the facts, and discussed both with your doctor, it doesn't matter which path you choose, as long as all paths lead off the bench, and back into the game. Make a decision, commit, be strong, follow through, and keep your eye on the prize.

So, congratulations on your new journey! For some of you it will be weight loss surgery, for others it will be a new way of eating or an exercise regime, and for some it will be a combination of strategies. It really does not matter. You *can* love yourself and still have aspects of you that you want to change. That's perfectly acceptable. The most important part of this journey is to find peace, health, and life, and to learn to accept and embrace yourself for the fabulous and valuable human being you are. Demand nothing less from yourself, or others.

Always, always, always, remember to laugh ... it's Botox® for the soul!

Judith Brown Clarke

Judi was born in Milwaukee, Wisconsin, moved to Kokomo, Indiana, and finished her childhood in Lansing, Michigan. She is married to husband, Hugh, and is the mother of three wonderful sons: Dorian – age 19, Mychael – age 18, and Antonio – age 8. She is also the proud owner of Chance the dog, and Sponge Bob the fish.

She holds two degrees from Michigan State University, a Bachelor of Science in Audiology & Speech Science, and a Master of Education degree. She is currently completing her doctoral dissertation for her Ph.D. in Public Administration and Public Policy from Western Michigan University, from which she will graduate with honors. In addition to working for the State of Michigan, and attending to her family and dissertation, St. Paul's Episcopal Church in Lansing, Michigan, has her unconditional and total devotion.

Judi has experienced athletic success in the 400-Meter Hurdle event as a five-time National Champion, and Silver Medalist in the 1984 Olympic Games in Los Angeles, California. She has held numerous National and World Records, and still owns an as yet unbroken World Record as a member of the distance medley relay team in which she ran the 400-Meter leg.

In addition, Judi was a three time Gold Medalist at the Pan-American Games, was a Silver Medalist at the World Track and Field Championships, and was a twelve time Big Ten Champion in Track and Field events. In 1986 she was inducted into the Michigan State University Hall of Fame, and in 1987 she was named as one of the "Athletes of the Year," specifically "Sportswoman of the Year" by Sports Illustrated™ magazine. Judi has also been honored by having carried the Olympic torch on its tour across America.

Judi has been a Big Ten Track and Field Coach, and a sought after, nationally recognized motivational speaker working with corporations, civic groups, and schools across the country. Her current civic responsibilities include membership on the Ingham County Women's Commission, and participating in other good works sponsored by her church.

The jump is so frightening

between where I am

and where I want to be...

because of all I may

become

I will close my eyes

and leap!

MARY ANNE RADMACHER

Welcome to the weird, wild, wonderful world of weight loss surgery! Whether you're just here for a brief visit to get the lay of the land, or you intend to make this your permanent home, we're here to answer your questions and show you around. We're the Welcome Wagon, of sorts.

In fact showing you around is exactly what this book is about. This book is for those of you who are considering having a weight loss procedure done, as well as for those of you who have already made the decision to have surgery and are at various stages in the process. We wrote this book for all the REAL people out there who need information on more than just the medical facts (although we provide that as well). This book is written BY REAL PEOPLE, FOR REAL PEOPLE.

We're not celebrities (except in our own minds...), and we don't have private chefs to cook our meals for us, personal trainers to help us work out, or live celebrity jet-set lifestyles. We don't have therapists on speed dial, plastic surgeons on retainer, or an endless supply of time and money to shop for clothes every time we lose weight. We're the working stiffs who have to do this by ourselves, and work it all in around spouses, kids, jobs, school, chores, friends, and everything else. We're the people who have real life to deal with every day, while we try to find a way to just have a "life," let alone a happy and healthy one.

The purpose of this book is to tell it like it is. In a way, it's sort of a glimpse into a "day-in-the-life" of two ordinary women from Michigan. We're not sugarcoating anything, and we leave it to you to decide whether you want to experience the same things we do or not. We're not going to tell you that with weight loss surgery you can "have it all!" Maybe you will, maybe you won't. But then maybe you'll hit the lottery tonight too.... Some people have this surgery and do end up looking like stars, models, and "celeb-utantes." For the other 99.9% of us, however, here's what life is like on a daily basis: sometimes funny, sometimes a little painful, but always totally real.

We're not going to tell you our life histories in this book, nor use it as a forum for working through all of our personal pain and angst from years gone by. This book isn't about how ripped off and hard-done-by we were, it's about what you can really expect if you make the decision to change your life through weight loss surgery. It's about how we came to the decision to do so, and what we've experienced since making that decision.

Our intent is to provide you with useful and practical information about the types of surgeries being done today, the risks and benefits of them, and about what you might experience as a result of having surgery to help you lose weight. If you haven't yet made the decision, then our purpose here is to give you as much useful and applicable information as we can to help you decide whether this is the right direction for you, and if it is, to give you the information necessary to help you find a surgeon who will take good and proper care of you.

To assist you with that, we've included for your consideration the good, the bad, the yukky, and the strange. We've tried not to oversimplify anything, while still making it easy to understand. Some of you have already learned a bit about weight loss surgery, while others are learning about it for the first time. If you're in the advanced group, please be patient for the sake of the beginners. Hopefully the stories will be helpful, or at least keep you amused.

You read the information and the stories, and *you* determine what weight to give them in making your decision (no pun intended). In fact, while you're reading we suggest that you make a pro/con list to help you make your decision. No one can make this decision for you, and no one knows what's scary or appealing to you, but you. So, as you read along, if something either strikes you as a very negative aspect of surgery, or a very positive aspect of surgery, write it down on your decision list for later reference.

Similarly, if you have questions that arise as you read, and you can't find the answers in the book, make a list of questions as you think of them, and tuck them in the back of the book. You can then take the book, your deicsion list, and your notes to a physician ('cause we will tell you how to find a good one!), and efficiently get the answers to all your questions and concerns.

Speaking of what you can't find in this book, you won't find recipes, or exercise routines, insurance information, or tax benefits. For information on those issues, we suggest (in respective order), consulting your mother or aunt, the guy in the tight t-shirt and shorts at the gym, the human resource person at your job, and an accountant that gives a free consultation to new clients. In that vein, and as we tell the college students we teach, Julie is *a* lawyer, but she's not *your* lawyer, so please don't send email with legal questions.

What you will find in this book is information on what to do if you start to lose your hair after surgery (see Chapter Six), experiences that are particular only to men (see Chapter Ten), tips and tricks from people who've been down the path before you, a heads-up on things to avoid, and a really serious discussion about whether or not you should even read this book. We've assembled some pretty awesome people to talk to you about the technical stuff, and we made sure to pick people who have a good sense of humor so you won't be bored.

We tried to keep the book on an upbeat note, but there are certain topics or stories that just require a more serious tone. We do not intend to make light of the serious nature of having surgery, nor do we intend to treat lightly the issues with which bariatric patients must deal. What we do intend, however, is to drive home the fact that you have to keep your sense of humor, something in which we wholeheartedly believe.

As for the layout of the book, since there is more than one voice being communicated in each chapter, we had to pick a head spokesperson for each one. So, when you are reading along, the first name that appears in the list of authors for that chapter is who's doing the talking for the group – unless we explicitly tell you otherwise. (Just like a lawyer to have a loophole built in....) The other authors have contributed their thoughts, ideas, and information, but realistically, only one person can talk at a time. You'll note that a majority of the time it's Julie speaking. How fitting that we should choose a lawyer/college professor to be our mouthpiece.

Because all of us are prone to using big, obscure, or technical words, for your convenient reference we've included a glossary of terms in the back of the book. (We realize there's just never a dictionary around when you need one….) To keep the page count down, and thus the cost of the book, we only printed the most important terms in the book glossary. A more comprehensive glossary is available, however, for free download on our web site which is listed in the front of the book. Also, if you'd like more information on certain topics, we've provided a list of web sites and other sources for you, again we've included the most important ones and put the rest on the web site for you to download at no charge.

We've included all the research sources used to write this book, but many of the other resources we would like to have published were just going to drive up the cost of the book. We didn't want to do that because we know you have other, more important things on which to spend your money. So check out the web site, because there's a number of great things there to see, read, download, or print for free. Call it our little gift to you.

Well, that's about it for all the stuff we think you might need to know before you take your wild ride through the world of weight loss surgery. We hope you find it informative, helpful, insightful, and a little fun. Keep smiling, and remember you are not alone. You have the power to change your life by whatever means necessary.

The two most important things

I did learn were that you are as powerful

and strong as you allow yourself to be,

and that the most difficult part of any endeavor

is taking the first step,

making the first decision.

ROBYN DAVIDSON

Chapter One

⟜ R E A L I T Y S L A P ! ! ⟞

Julie M. Janeway
Karen J. Sparks

Well, before we start on this journey, we need to sit down and have a big emotional heart-to-heart about some things. You'll need to do a little soul searching at this point. If you're a woman reading this, you are no doubt ready for such an event. If you're a man, well as I tell my husband, just suck it up and deal with it.

First things first: Do not do this for anyone else but you. If you choose to begin down this path, you must be one hundred percent honest with yourself about why you're doing this, and for whom you are doing it. You must come to grips with who you are now, and how you got this way.

Although there are many contributing factors that help people gain weight, the reality is you got here by putting the food in your mouth all by yourself. Ultimately you are responsible for what went in, and what will go in your mouth in the future. You are in control of how you maintain your health and live your life. You have chosen the paths you've taken, and you, alone, will navigate new roads in the future.

You must choose to start down this road solely to take as much control over your life, weight, and food as you had over gaining the weight and eating the food thus far. You must be doing it for your own health, and control of your own life. You must be doing it to stay alive, and to be able to directly and meaningfully participate in life. You must want to create for yourself a new healthy life and lifestyle that will allow you to do what you want, and be in control of where you want to go. You must do this to please you.

You cannot do this to please anyone else, or in hopes of changing the nature of any relationships in your life. This must be a totally selfish act. Although this act must be completely about you, it is okay for it to have derivative benefits for others. The most direct and important benefits must, however, relate solely to you.

If you are thinking of undertaking this endeavor so you can give more to your children, or your spouse, or your career, then you need to stop and re-think your motives. This endeavor must be about being in control of yourself, about feeling emotionally and physically strong, and about living to see your next birthday. These are the primary reasons and direct benefits of such an undertaking. Secondary benefits may accrue in that you will be around longer and be able to interact more with your children and spouse, but don't make them the primary purpose of the event.

Undertaking this act has to be about hitting bottom, and from the very depths of your being, truly wanting to give up this painful existence. You have to be willing to literally reinvent yourself, and you can't do that if you're not focusing on you. If you're focusing on the needs or wants of others with regard to your weight, or because you think that your weight is the only thing standing in the way of all your dreams coming true, then think again.

This process is not just about losing weight, it's about molding and re-shaping a whole new existence. It isn't just about an incision, or a medical procedure, or numbers on a scale. It's about metamorphosis. If all you're ready to do is fight your way out of the cocoon, and not undergo the long, arduous, and amazing change from being one creature to becoming another, then you need to stop and re-examine your choices. If you are willing to undergo this process of transformation, then you must now examine your expectations and anticipated outcomes, and gauge them against reality.

Reality (in case you are laboring under this massive misconception), rarely, if ever resembles anything you see on television – not even on the Discovery Channel®. The ordinary and mundane don't bring ratings and high paying sponsors. The unusual and exceptional are the mainstays of television viewership.

Many of you reading this book have watched one or more television shows documenting the life of a bariatric surgery patient. Whether it be on a talk show, or on the Discovery Health Channel®, we've all seen these amazing stories of transfiguration, white knights, true love, and dreams come true. We've all seen the people who've lost 350 or more pounds and gone from a size 38 to a 4, or from a 10x shirt to a men's large. We've heard them tell us of finding true love, of becoming championship athletes, of going from being a nobody to being a cover model for a health and fitness magazine. And those stories are for the most part true, but for every one of those people who has experienced such a one-in-ten-million experience, there's ten million who've just experienced real life.

All the people who go through this process, who just experience their daily lives (albeit in a happier and healthier way), aren't the people that talk shows and documentary producers generally care about. They're not interesting television fare because they're just you and me.

These ordinary people are the ones who lose a lot of weight, but they still wear a regular size, they still have body issues they don't like, they don't end up on a magazine cover, and they may still be looking for a decent person with whom to have a relationship and share their life. Worse, maybe their relationship blew up because they lost so much weight and took the time to focus on themselves. That's not good television. It hits too close to home for many viewers. People think,"I can see that in my own family room. Thanks, but no thanks."

Reality is that you might go from a size 32 to a 14, not a 4. Reality is going from a 60 inch waist to a 38, not a 30. Reality is feeling better, and stronger, and being healthier, not becoming famous. Reality is you don't get younger, although you may look younger. Reality is you'll probably have some flabby skin, and you'll still have problem areas that you hate on your body, not that you'll become a championship athlete or a cover model. Reality is that stuff starts going south about age 35. Reality is if you had a crappy marriage before you lost weight, chances are you'll still have a crappy marriage after. But reality is also that you will still be as worthy of a great life and the chance to live it as those people who experienced the unique and unusual.

The reality is this is not a magic pill, or a cure-all. Weight loss surgery doesn't guarantee a great life; it only gives you the opportunity to live a happier, healthier, and hopefully longer life. Ultimately, you still determine whether or not you have a great life. You make those choices, and you choose whether or not to fix other broken areas of your life. You choose, not anybody else.

You will still have to deal with the garbage that comes your way, and you still determine how you live your life and whether it's worth living. Everything doesn't turn to gold just because you lose the weight. What does happen is you may find you have the ability to, and the inspiration to make it better, or to make a change; to make gold out of straw if you will. Deal with that concept and you're well on your way to dealing with not being a fat person any more.

So we've got you thinking about all this painful stuff, and you think you can wrap your head around transforming your life. You believe you can do this for you, and you can have realistic expectations about the outcome. But can you deal with the fact that although you may change the weight, the appearance, and the lifestyle, you can never change the emotional memories and scars of being fat?

It's true. They never go away, but you can learn to control them and no longer let them control you. You'll always feel some pain from past rejections, missed opportunities and events, lost chances and hurtful remarks, but you don't need to live in fear of them anymore either.

You'll confront these emotional monsters, every last one of them, at least ten times throughout this process. You'll feel the pain of each one over and over again. Eventually, you'll learn to control them and realize that they're in the past, and you control the future. In contrast, you'll experience the thrills of each new victory at least ten times over as well. If you're willing to wade through this morass of emotional issues and ride the proverbial emotional roller coaster in order to get it behind you for good, then stand up and take the next step down the road to a new life.

Your new life starts with knowing yourself physically and emotionally, and being ready to make the changes needed to keep yourself alive and healthy. This self-examination will also come in handy when you hear stories about medical complications, or people who put their weight back on, or people who encountered a host of other obstacles. Remembering that you are unique physiologically, psychologically, and emotionally will help you to remember that other people's problems and issues aren't necessarily going to be your problems and issues. If you can be prepared to deal with what comes your way, or doesn't, then take another step down the road. As they say, prepare for the worst, and hope for the best.

Preparing for the worst and hoping for the best includes doing your research. In reading this book, you're doing both. It is unbelievably important for you to know what you're getting into, both medically and emotionally. You need to be fully medically informed as to your options, your limitations, the benefits, and the risks of having a bariatric procedure done. You need to fully understand all the science behind what is being undertaken, and you need to be aware of the percentage of incidence of each type of foreseeable complication.

Also, be cognizant of the fact that there can be unforeseen complications due to the unique nature of your physiology, and just because one person had thus and such, doesn't mean you'll have it too. Karen had to have her gallbladder out three months after her surgery, and I had a post-operative stricture three different times. Just because she had one type of complication didn't mean I would have it also, and vice versa. Neither instance was the fault of the surgeon, but both are known complications or after-effects of the procedure.

Complications happen. If you have one, just deal with it and move on. It doesn't mean the doctor messed up; it's just a complication derived from opening up the body and reconstructing it. It may not be a nice situation, and you may not feel like dealing with it. That's normal, but you get through it.

What is not normal is to assume the doctor made a mistake. As a lawyer myself, (and I can't believe I'm saying this...), don't run off to see an attorney if you have complications from this surgery. If you have complications not remotely associated with this type of surgery (like you're missing your left kidney afterward...), then maybe consult a lawyer. Other than that, just concentrate on getting through it with your doctor's help.

When doing your research you need to be looking at facilities and surgeons that will give you a lot of information. If you are dealing with organizations and individuals who simply want to get your insurance card and book you a surgery date, *run*, don't walk the other way. Don't play bariatric roulette with your life.

Respectable and reputable organizations should be providing a full orientation that offers detailed information on the procedure, and the risks and benefits. It should also provide substantial pre-operative medical evaluation and testing by both an internist and a surgeon to determine whether or not the patient is a medically sound candidate for surgery, and whether or not laparoscopic procedures can or should be used.

Additionally, good bariatric surgical centers require a psychological assessment of the potential patient to determine whether the patient is emotionally able to withstand the process, is going into the process with the right motivations, and whether the person has reasonable and rational expectations of the process and themselves. Good treatment centers also usually require an assessment of the significant support person in the patient's life to determine whether the patient will have proper and adequate emotional support throughout the process, and to determine whether situations may exist that will sabotage or undermine the patient's success.

Having a good support system is critical to bariatric patients. Although you must do it for yourself, you can't do it alone. There's just too much to deal with. You need people who will listen, even if they don't really understand what you're going through. They need to be people who will help you see the positive in the unknowns ahead of you, not tell you that the light at the end of the tunnel is an oncoming train. You need to have people who will love you no matter how you look, or how you change.

My husband, family, and friends were a constant source of support for me, as were Karen's family and friends. They supported us, but they didn't really understand what we were going through. Karen and I went through this process together, and without each other neither one of us would have made it because only we understood what the other was going through. Good support is the key to success, both in your personal life, and in your surgeon's office.

Persons seeking bariatric treatment should also require that their surgeon's office provide nutritional and exercise counseling, as well as be affiliated with other surgeons who are trained to handle particular bariatric related complications, or other matters if necessary. Surgeons should also provide extensive follow-up care, and patients should be ready and willing to attend all follow up appointments, have all testing done, and follow through on the process. Surgeons should be prepared to deal with a number of issues that may follow surgery, not simply tell the patient to seek treatment from a primary care physician.

Incidentally, primary care physicians should not be solely responsible for the treatment of obesity related conditions such as high blood pressure or diabetes. These types of conditions are intricately entwined in the surgical and weight loss process, and should be monitored and attended to by the surgeon and internist in consultation with the patient's primary care or other appropriate physician. Bariatric surgery has a proven track record of effectively dealing with conditions such as high blood pressure and diabetes, and Dr. Baker will address this issue in Chapter Three.

Dr. Baker will also discuss the length of the process, and why it should not be rushed. I've personally been appalled at some of the documentaries I've seen on T.V. that showed patients having massive reconstructive plastic surgery within ten months of their bariatric surgery. At ten months your body is still losing weight and adjusting to its new form. Your skin and muscle haven't been given enough time to shrink as far as they might be able to go without surgical intervention. Perhaps the skin won't shrink back all the way, but maybe a less drastic cosmetic surgical procedure could be used if so much skin weren't being removed.

This is a process that simply can't be rushed. It operates on its own time schedule, and each patient's body responds at a different rate. But I seriously doubt that the body of anyone who loses 150+ pounds in ten months has finished adjusting in that time frame.

Because it is a lengthy process, potential surgery candidates must be prepared to be patient and compliant. Trust me when I say, it really works best if you listen to what they tell you and follow the instructions. They don't just tell you this stuff for the good of their health – in fact, they tell you for the good of your health!

Now, I admit to the fact that I am a person who needs to push and test the limits because I know that I'm a unique individual, and I don't necessarily respond physically the same way everyone else does. So when they told me not to drink orange juice, I ran right out and drank orange juice. Six hours later when I got up off the bathroom floor, I decided they were right and I shouldn't drink orange juice. It's not that you can never have orange juice again, but maybe you just shouldn't slam half a glass of orange juice three months after surgery. Just a theory....

So the point of that story (and later on you'll read so many more) is to trust in the doctors' expertise, follow their guidance and instructions, and commit yourself to the process body and soul – literally. Remind yourself that you are learning entirely new skills, and learning skills effectively means practicing them over and over. Practice your new skills of controlling your food, your health, and your lifestyle.

By the way, if you think that food controlled you before your surgery, you ain't seen nothing yet! Once you have this surgery, food will control you like never before; but in a good way. I say that because unlike smokers or drinkers, we can't just stop eating to rid ourselves of the problem (and yes, I know quitting smoking or drinking is incredibly difficult. Don't send any hate mail !!)

We must eat to survive, and we must eat well to be healthy and thrive, but because of the nature of this surgery, you need to eat more often each day than you probably did, eat less food at one sitting than you probably ever did, and eat only certain kinds of foods while staying away from others. Timing, proportions, food types, and access to acceptable foods becomes a serious challenge.

Coping with this challenge is the biggest new skill you'll master. Every single day is a new adventure. We'll talk about this later in Chapter Twelve entitled "The Protein Safari." Learning these new food skills is unbelievably important because if you don't, and you fall back into your old habits, you can put the weight back on. You will have gone through all of this for absolutely nothing. Don't go there.

In fact, you need to be comfortable with the fact that if you begin this journey it's a one way trip. What you'll shed along the way will be more than just pounds, and the person who concludes the journey will only resemble on the inside the person who started it.

You must be comfortable with change, and willing to conquer fear. In fact, when both Karen and I wrestled with the decision to begin down this path, we came to rely on the wise words of my sister Cheryl. She reminded us, as we've many times since reminded each other: "You can do anything afraid, that you can do unafraid."

The person who travels this road has to know they can face fear, as well as fear of the unknown. The person who starts this journey has to want to participate in life. The person who walks this path has to want to live life and take advantage of what it has to offer. The person who takes these steps has to be ready to leave a lot of pain behind and happily face the future. The person who begins this process has to want to go through the metamorphosis that will make them grateful for who they are and always have been on the inside, and finally grateful for who they have become on the outside.

Now ask yourself: "Am I that person?"

If you are that person, then you're ready to read the rest of this book. In fact, read it twice!

Welcome to the rest of your life.

Chapter Two

➤ E N - L I G H T E N M E N T ➤

Julie M. Janeway
Karen J. Sparks

If you're reading this you must at least be willing to change your life through weight loss surgery, and are ready to find out more about it in order to make a really informed decision. Congratulations on getting this far!

We've named this chapter "En-Lightenment" because that's what it is truly about: being enlightened intellectually and emotionally regarding the procedure and process of weight loss through surgery, as well as the en-"lightenment" of losing a large amount of weight, and ridding yourself of a lot of the emotional load you carry as part and parcel of being overweight. With that being said, we think it prudent to tell you a little bit about the authors of this book, as we are going to be your guides through portions of your investigation and enlightenment process. We also thought you might like to know a bit about what brought Karen and me to the decision to change our lives, and be rid of the weight forever.

JULIE

My name is Julie Janeway, and for as long as I can remember I was overweight. Not just overweight, but until high school, always the tallest kid in school too. Like you, I tried every diet under the sun, and a few of them even worked for a short while. But, the weight always came back – with a vengeance! Although I wasn't happy with the fact that I was overweight, I just always assumed that it was my lot in life, and God must have made me that way for a reason.

I spent my life like most overweight kids, being teased, being picked on, always wanting to fit in, but always a little on the periphery of things socially. I missed out on a lot of things in life because of my weight, but my mother did her utmost to help me diet, teach me to like and respect myself, and make sure that I had whatever I needed to feel and look like the other kids, even if it was only a reasonable facsimile of what they had.

If a particular brand of jeans were the "in" thing, and they weren't made in my size, my mom would take me wherever I needed to go to find something close, but in a plus size. Every store on the hunt, however, was a serious and painful reminder that I couldn't just go where everybody else went to buy those jeans.

Whether or not I could wear the "in" jeans of the moment, I was an intelligent, quick-witted, extrovert in high school, and I didn't lack for friends or school activities to attend. No matter how much I tried to believe I was just like everybody else, I always knew I wasn't like everybody else because of my weight.

My intelligence and wit set me apart somewhat, but my weight was always the true dividing line between "them" and "me." I've asked a million times if I've asked once, "Why am I like this, and they're not?" Maybe I was meant to be overweight in order to force me to focus my life on other things, like education, or helping others, or advocating for others who were disenfranchised from society. Blah, blah, blah…fill in the blank with whatever reason you can think of because no doubt you've had this conversation in your head a zillion times too.

I thought getting a good education would help me feel better about myself, and it did, to a certain extent. I earned an Associate degree in Business, a Bachelor of Business degree (with four minors!), a Law degree (Magna Cum Laude), a Master degree in Business, and am now finishing my dissertation on my Ph.D. in Public Administration and Public Policy. Although I am very proud of the fact that I put myself through school on my own dime, and pulled top grades while working a full time job, it still didn't put me right in the center of the zip code for Normal, U.S.A. In fact, if anything, it put me further away.

Do I regret getting my education? No! Knowledge is power! But, I was resigned to the fact that I was a heavy girl with a lot of education and a sharp sense of humor, and that just made me radically different from the rest of the world for many, many reasons. I figured that was how I was supposed to be, and I needed to accept it.

I was learning to accept it the best I could, but I never liked it – no, not one bit. Even after law school, I kept trying to lose weight and stay active, as owning your own law firm keeps you hopping. I was always on the hunt for another diet that might be the magic formula for me. I had never even entertained the thought of weight loss surgery, and then April 26, 2001, appeared on the calendar, and life as I knew it changed forever.

That day, I was scheduled to be in three different cities over the day. When I came back to my office after the second court appearance, I was talking to my paralegal about not wanting to drive across the state to appear at this city council hearing as I just had a bad feeling about it. I didn't really feel like it had anything to do with the hearing, I just sort of felt this impending sense of doom. My hearing was at 7:30 p.m., and by 3:30 p.m., I was actually starting to feel a little queasy about going. I even mentioned something to my paralegal, and she assured me I was just tired from driving around the state all day.

So away I went with my paralegal's voice echoing in my head that I was just tired out. As I was driving through Grand Rapids (I live in Michigan), traffic started to pick up, and I knew I'd hit rush hour. It was 5:50 p.m., and not only was it rush hour, it was happy hour too. I changed lanes from the right to the left to allow for the traffic merging onto the highway.

I noticed a brand new black Sunfire coming up the on-ramp very fast. I noticed it partly because it was moving so fast, but also because I'd been looking at buying one just days before. This particular Sunfire had completely blacked out windows, and I noticed that because completely blacked out windows are illegal in Michigan. I carried on my merry way, slowing to about 72 miles per hour in the left lane (traffic speed), and assumed all was as it should be. The black Sunfire had the entire empty right lane in which to merge, and I thought that would be that. Wrong!

The Sunfire merged into the right lane, and then decided that it had to immediately be in the left lane, and swerved directly in front of me, clipping the right front corner of my car. The hit shoved me onto the gravel shoulder of the road. I tried to correct the swerve, but the car was now sliding sideways on the gravel, and that was all she wrote folks! The car rolled twice, then went end over end, and then rolled two more times before sliding to a stop on its roof on the shoulder of the right lane of the road.

As the car began to flip over I stiffened and braced myself, and then something told me to relax or I'd end up breaking every bone in my body. So I went limp, and went for the ride of my life. After the first roll, the driver side window smashed out, and the seatbelt fixture ripped away from the wall of the car. I was no longer strapped in, so I was thrown around pretty good. At one point I was even in the back seat! As I was being tossed about, I distinctly remember thinking that this must be what running shoes feel like when they're in the dryer!

Unfortunately as the car rolled and skidded, my left leg got out the driver side smashed window, and it got pretty badly crushed. Much of my lower leg was actually missing, but I didn't know it at that time. I just remember feeling it scraping along the road, and using all my energy to lift my leg up and away from the road because I thought, "That's not good…."

The amazing thing about my accident is that not one other car hit me as I rolled in front of a pretty heavy flow of traffic on Interstate 96 at rush hour. People ran to help, and I tried to determine whether I was dead or alive. I reasoned that if I could actually have that conversation in my head, I must be alive. (I think, therefore I am…) I tried to sit up (I was now laying on the roof of the car because it was upside down), and my back was pretty sore. I remember thinking, "Oh man! I'm going to end up looking like a human question mark for at least a week over this! I've seriously pulled some muscles!"

Despite the pain in my back, I sat up anyway, and noticed all the glass around me. I didn't seem to be bleeding, so I guessed I was okay. I quickly noticed that the entire dashboard had come out of the car, and virtually nothing was where it should be. There were no windows left, the center armrest was in the back seat, and what was left of my cell phone was a tangled and melted mess.

Then I remembered my leg, and how it had been dragging on the pavement. Strangely, I couldn't feel any pain, so I thought it must just be a little cut or something. I pulled myself up far enough to look at it, and as soon as I saw it, I thought two things: "Oh crap, that's probably going to require surgery," and "Huh, fat really is yellow."

Then the pain hit me. It hit so hard that I thought the car had been hit by a semi-truck. I laid back down and just began screaming because it was the only thing I knew to do. The pain was excruciating, but somehow it confirmed for me that I was alive. People came to help, police and fire trucks eventually arrived, and I was taken to Spectrum Hospital in Grand Rapids.

Spectrum Hospital is a level one regional trauma center, and a fantastic hospital. To make a long story short (because that's another book entirely), they took phenomenal care of me for the months I spent there recovering. They saved my leg, they treated my broken back (three vertebrae and three squashed discs), and they saved my life. I'll always be eternally grateful.

So how does all this relate to this book? Well here's how it came to be. Because my leg was almost completely destroyed in the accident, they gave me little chance of keeping it. Three inches of the bone was missing for crying out loud, not to mention most of the muscles were gone. Besides all the medication and surgeries (one every second day for over a month), they said I had to be plied with as much calcium and nutrition as they could get into me to keep the bone and tissues alive.

I could have cared less about eating while I was in the hospital because I was so stoked-out on Morphine and other pain killers, plus being constantly doped up with anesthetic to go into surgery, so food was not on the priority list. They force-fed me almost, and I hated every second of it.

When I came home from the hospital, I was still completely bed-bound, and I had 'round the clock nurses and caregivers who were instructed to get as much calcium and other nutrients into me as humanly possible. By that time, I was so stinking sick of somebody trying to shove ice cream in my face, I thought I'd become homicidal! I remember pleading that I didn't want any more cheese, or milkshakes, or ice cream because I was going to put on more weight, and how would I get it off?

They told me to worry about saving my leg now, and worry about getting rid of the fat later. All fine and good if you're not on the fat end of the stick! So on the pounds went over those two and a half years of recovery. Ten, twenty, forty, eighty, a hundred pounds. Arrrgggghhhhh…..!!!!! I cringe just thinking about it! I was heavy to begin with, I didn't need any more weight. Especially when they kept telling me I would never walk again. I was determined to walk again, and I was determined to get that stupid weight off me. After all, I didn't even get to enjoy putting it on!

So I told my amazing orthopedic surgeon, Dr. John Stubbart, (the man who helped save my leg), that I was thinking about having gastric bypass surgery done, because now I was so heavy I couldn't even get out of the wheelchair by myself. I told him that I was determined to *walk* down the aisle to marry my fiance Matt, and I wasn't going to spend my married life fat, or in a wheelchair!

I also talked to him about my medical concerns, not the least of which was yet another surgery and more scars. He told me about Dr. Randal Baker and the Michigan Medical P.C.®, Center for Health Excellence. He told me that not only were they highly qualified and experienced surgeons, but they did the gastric bypass procedure laparoscopically, so it wasn't as invasive a surgery. Less invasive means less scars, and to me that was a better option because I'd had enough invasive surgery, and the lower half of me looks like a map drawn by Rand-McNally!

So off I went to see Dr. Baker, and the rest is history. I started at 368 pounds, and was a size 28. Now I'm down 177 pounds and am a size 14. I walk very well thank you very much, and my leg and back are profoundly glad I did it.

Just prior to having my surgery, however, I went back to work at a new college as a professor, and met my new boss Karen Sparks, Dean of Business Administration and Technology. We became immediate friends, almost on sight. We were kindred spirits in more ways than one.

And with that, I think now is a good time for Karen to introduce herself to you. So, here, in her own words is Karen to tell you about how she came to the decision to have weight loss surgery.

KAREN

Hello, my name is Karen Sparks. I'm going to tell you about how I came to have weight loss surgery, but to do that entails telling you a little about my life, as I didn't have any one particular defining moment or event that caused me to make the decision. Instead, it was the culmination of a lifetime of events that lead me to a surgical solution. I'm not afraid to say that what you're about to read was pretty hard for me to dredge up and face again. It was very hard to write, but for better or worse, and as painful as it is, here we go....

I have been heavy all of my life. Even as a very young child I knew I was different. Fat, heavy, big boned, chubby, what ever you want to call it, that was me. I've spent an incalculable amount of time in my life asking, "Why did I have to be this way?" or "Why me?" As far back as I can remember, I just wanted to be normal.

From grade school through high school, I just wanted to be like everyone else. I watched as my sister picked out cute clothes from about any store we visited. My options were limited to the "chubby girls" section at Sears or Montgomery Ward. Christmas after Christmas came and went wherein I received clothes that always had to be returned; the clothes never fit, no matter the good intentions. Christmas after Christmas came and went with me putting on a brave and happy face to cover the disappointment, embarrassment, and pain of not being normal.

Disappointment and embarrassment weren't limited to Christmas though. I never got invited to birthday parties, sleepovers, school dances, or the prom. I constantly had to hide my disappointment with a laissez-faire attitude, and half a loaf of bread and butter helped soothe the pain a bit too. Countless hours were spent crying in silence and solitude on the floor in the back of my closet.

Always an outsider, the only thing that allowed me to be a part of things was my art, a good sense of humor, and the fact that I was smart. Everyone knew that "Sparky" could draw. No one could compete with me on that, and they knew it. "Sparky" was funny, she could always take a joke, no matter how pointed or mean it might be. And "Sparky" was smart. She always had the answers, and was willing to teach others how to find them when need be. That was how I participated: on the fringe of things with a smile on my face.

I was a participant only in the background, in the shadows where I didn't have to worry about being seen, but I desperately wanted to be seen. I watched as my older brother and sister went to dances and the prom, and out on weekend dates with their boyfriends and girlfriends. I watched as they picked out the special clothes and other things that come along with the rites of passage through your teen years, and I faced the pain of knowing that somehow I would never get to share in those experiences.

Later, came my younger brother following the same path of "normal" childhood activities, special memories, and events. Instead of "normal" childhood and adolescent activities, I spent my time with my books and my drawings. I played in the school band because it was a place where I could be a part of something "normal." But still, I sat too many hours on the floor in my closet crying and asking my mom, "When will it be my turn?" "Why do I have to be this way?" "Will there ever be anyone for me?" "What did I do to deserve this?" And many, many other questions she could never answer.

I spent the greater part of my school years just wanting people to like me, and trying desperately to be like everyone else; or at least convince myself I was like everyone else. Deep in my heart I knew though, it was not going to happen for me because I wasn't "normal," and I wasn't thin.

There, too, was the pain of sitting in the kitchen with mom anxiously trying to help me in any way that she could to "diet." I distinctly remember sitting at the kitchen table at age 12 one summer day eating the tuna fish and cottage cheese mom had prepared for my lunch, as once again, we were trying to lose weight. I remember too many of those days throughout my life. I kept wishing there was a way to just lose the weight forever. Later that year, I found what I thought was my great white hope.

My first knowledge of weight-loss surgery was as early as 1970, during my 7th grade year of Jr. High. At that time, I read in the local paper of a doctor who was performing stomach stapling surgery in Hudson, not too far from my hometown of Jonesville, Michigan. I knew my parents would never be able to afford it, nor would they most likely ever even consider letting me go through the surgery at such a young age. Too young to pursue the program, I pushed it to the back of my mind with all my other hopes and dreams, and suffered with my weight problems through junior high and high school.

After high school I buried myself with work, two, sometimes three jobs at a time. I spent my money in ways that I hoped would make people like me. Instead of clothes and vacations with girlfriends, I bought tens of thousands of dollars worth of ornaments and collectibles. I spent my spare time always being the one to make things better for everyone else -- the fix-it person, despite my own wants and needs. There never seemed to be anyone making it better for me though. Why was I so alone, and so different?

At one time I did briefly drop 100 lbs over a summer, but I did it in a very unhealthy way. I was taking diet pills by the handful, and the weight just dropped off. As soon as I stopped taking the drugs, however, I immediately put the weight back on plus another 150 lbs. I was terrified that my weight would never stop going up. It seemed to me that it didn't matter what I ate, it simply made me gain weight. I was losing the fight, and I couldn't get an answer to the question, "Why?"

In trying to find that answer, there comes a point where you rationalize that God made you this way for a reason. Was I destined always just to be there to help everyone else get through their lives and be happy? Was I destined to be the rock and the make-it-better person for everyone else? Maybe so. But if that was true, what did I get out of the deal? I decided that what I got must be something to make me feel better, while helping to fix everyone else's life – an education.

I decided to go to college when I was thirty-two hoping that would change things for me. Unfortunately, no matter how educated you are the "fat prejudice" still follows you around. Because of that, social situations didn't change much at college. Still, going to school became a passion, as I could be noticed for being smart there, but it held little consolation for the events to which I was not invited, was too old, or was simply forgotten about. Overall, it was no different than my previous school years. Why I thought it would be different, I don't know.

I may not have been the life of the party while at college, but I did earn a Bachelor degree in Business Administration, and went on for a Master degree in Business Education. I'd acquired the degrees, and I had the intelligence, yet I didn't feel a bit more normal because of my weight.

As I once again searched for a way to lose weight (and I tried them all mind you), I came to the conclusion that I was forever destined to be overweight and never to be normal. I thought I could accept that, if it weren't for the part of me that knew that with all the science and discovery in our world, someone should be able to come up with something to help me. Why weren't they finding it? Why wasn't I finding it? Then I stumbled across the concept of weight loss surgery again.

Once I began to research weight loss surgery more seriously, I came to understand that there was help out there. How to get to it became my next hurdle. After five years of research, mounds of information from the Internet, and mailings from a multitude of organizations that were willing to do the job, I was just not satisfied with any of them. Those who were good enough by my standards weren't remotely close enough geographically. I began to get really discouraged.

To be truthful, it was during the summer of 2003, that I knew I had to do something about my weight, as I was dangerously close to being in serious trouble. At that time, my weight was at its highest, 425 lbs, and I was flirting carelessly with high blood pressure. I had been researching weight loss surgery with little success in finding a program I believed to be sound, and then came the day I met Julie Janeway.

I was the Dean of Business and Technology at a small college. Julie had sent me her resume looking for work as a professor, and I just happened to need someone with her credentials and experience. I knew we were destined to be friends from the first exchange of voicemail messages. It was Julie who shared with me her knowledge of Dr. Baker and the staff at MMPC® Center for Health Excellence in Grand Rapids, Michigan. That was a major turning point in my life. I was intrigued, if not a little wary, but I decided to find out the details.

I researched MMPC® and Dr. Baker, went to an orientation, had all my questions answered, came home satisfied, and a little scared. What I'd waited for, a permanent solution to my weight issues, was now staring me in the face. I struggled with the decision whether or not to go for it. In my head I could hear Julie's sister Cheryl telling me that I "could do anything afraid, that I could do unafraid." Believing in that, all I had to do was think about all I had missed in my life, and the decision was made.

When I had surgery I weighed 425 pounds, and was wearing a size 34 to 36. Now I have lost 225 pounds, and wear a size 14. I will never go back to where I was before. Just sitting down to write this is as much of that type of pain and heartache as I can bear, let alone actually having to relive it. I am a new person now, and I'm enjoying finding out who was hiding inside me all those years. I don't know if I could have done it alone, but Julie and I resolved to go through the process together, and together we'll help take you through it as well.

OUR SURGERIES

Karen and I went through our surgeries together…well sort of. I had my surgery done on October 29, 2003, which was the day after my birthday (Happy Birthday to me). I took a slot that was vacated by someone who had cancelled, and I only had eleven days notice. Immediately I went on the protein fast that you must complete before the surgery to shrink your liver, and went through a whirlwind of medical tests to make sure I was in good shape for a Roux-en-Y gastric bypass. I got through everything just Jim-Dandy-fine, and the next thing I knew I was there, and it was happening.

Karen lived through those first few weeks before and after surgery with me. She watched everything I went through during that time. She watched me trying to avoid food during that pre-op period, and she watched me get progressively more scared as the time neared. She helped me as best she could, and she made mental notes, because she was scheduled for the same surgery on December 12, 2003.

Karen had it a little tougher, pre-operatively speaking. She was on the protein fast for the full two weeks prior to surgery, which covered Thanksgiving. Thanksgiving with Karen's family is one of those affairs you see on T.V. It's kind of like an Osmond family reunion: tons of relatives, lots of food, happy happy. Karen loves these occasions, as she's such a family oriented person. It was extremely hard for her not to eat that day.

Additionally, Karen came home from the hospital the day before her birthday (which traditionally involves her family making her all her favorite foods), and she was still on the protein drink through Christmas and New Years! Never a braver soul have I met. The only consolation she had during these post-surgical times was that she really didn't give a rip whether or not she ate. Surgery does that to you.

But once we were both through the surgery, we kept each other afloat. We worked at making sure the other had eaten properly, had their water allotment, and taken their vitamins. We walked together, got sick together, and encouraged each other through plateaus. Despite a few rough patches that we'll discuss in later chapters, we made it through in fine style on the buddy system, and with the careful ministerings of Dr. Baker and his staff.

Dr. Baker, Dr. Foote, Dr. Kemmeter, and the rest of the staff at the MMPC® Center for Health Excellence in Grand Rapids, took extremely good care of us. In fact, every patient to whom we've spoken, has raved about the care they've received at this facility. As you search for a bariatric surgeon in your area, you should be expecting to find a surgeon who cares about you as an individual, and whose staff cares equally as much.

There are many first-rate bariatric surgeons across the country that utilize the multi-disciplinary approach to weight loss surgery. This entails the use of internal medicine specialists, behaviorists, dietitians, exercise physiologists, plastic surgeons, and of course trained bariatric (not just general) surgeons. We've included in the Additional Resources chapter a web site address for the American Society for Bariatric Surgery that has links to outstanding surgeons and bariatric medicine practices across the country to assist you in finding a practice that will take excellent care of you.

So you'll have an idea what to look for in a doctor, we'll kind of give you an introduction to our third co-author, Dr. Randal Baker. He's going to tell you a bit about why he became a bariatric surgeon, and then we'll sing his praises by relating to you a few of his fine qualities and credentials.

RANDAL S. BAKER, M.D., F.A.C.S.

So, how does one end up becoming a bariatric surgeon? I never remember waking up as a six-year-old boy declaring my intense desire to become a bariatric surgeon! In fact, after graduating from Calvin College in Grand Rapids, and Albany Medical College of New York, I never dreamed I would be involved in the battle against obesity. I had no significant exposure to bariatric surgery during medical school or residency, and planned for a quiet, hometown general surgical practice, with an emphasis in trauma and critical care.

During my Critical Care Fellowship, I did help treat several bariatric patients with significant complications who were sent to the Tertiary Care, Surgical Intensive Care Unit, but that was years before I ended up moving my practice into bariatric surgery. At the time, it didn't really pique my interest, maybe because I was only dealing with the intensive care portion of the process.

Several years later, after I became the Medical Director of the Surgical ICU and Assistant Director of the General Surgery Residency Program at Spectrum Hospital in Grand Rapids, Michigan, I was approached by one of our major HMOs to consider starting a bariatric surgical program. My practice group's physician medical practice already had a comprehensive, multi-disciplinary medical weight loss program (non-surgical). The HMO asked if we could develop a similar multidisciplinary approach to bariatric surgery. The request grew out of the fact that many surgical programs were offering no more than surgery, providing only tidbits of information, and lacking adequate pre-operative and post-operative care.

As I was plenty busy with trauma, critical care, general surgery, and my family (wife and seven children at this point), I was warned by other surgeons not to enter the bariatric arena, as it would completely engulf my practice, and encroach on all other elements. With the best of intentions, they also warned that morbidly obese patients were higher risk and can have significant complications, which can be taxing even for the most solid and laid back person. After much consideration and deliberation, however, and after about six months of continual prodding, the decision was made to create the surgical division of the MMPC® Weight Management Center.

To this day, I do not regret this decision at all. The bariatric practice did engulf my practice such that I stopped doing trauma, and other general surgery. Our center also had the opportunity to obtain two top-notch, caring surgeons in Dr. James Foote and Dr. Paul Kemmeter, both of whom were also trained in surgery and critical care. At times the trek has been trying and onerous, but I have no regrets.

In fact, I'm grateful for the course my professional life has taken. I have never had the opportunity to see such great benefits accrue in people's lives as a result of surgery, as I have with bariatric surgery. Words become insufficient in trying to relay the emotion I experience as patients go through a metamorphosis, and come back with tears in their eyes to describe their "new" world.

Emotion is also deep when patients experiencing complications or difficulty dealing with emotional issues go through trying times in an attempt to reach their "new" world. I can do the surgery, care for them medically, support them physically and emotionally, but I can't always make it better with a treatment or a prescription. I truly wish I could find a way to help even more.

As a result I have encouraged many of my patients to write a book about their weight loss surgery experiences, but to date, none of them had taken the challenge. Little did I know that two highly educated, motivated, and caring women would cross my path, and write what I consider to be the best-researched and written weight loss book on the market for the general public. This book is the "real deal," no sugar coated Hollywood fairy story here.

Although greater than 90% of bariatric patients experience no significant complications, it is important that patients recognize that complications do happen and can be significant in any surgery, including weight loss surgery. It so happens, however, that most bariatric complications are over "media-ized." Over a given period of time in a large hospital several patients may have complications and even die from joint replacement, or elective, general, and plastic surgery, or complications from obesity in general, yet it's the bariatric surgical cases that draw all the media attention. So don't buy into the media hype: just do your homework, weigh the risks, and make your own decision in consultation with your doctor.

Julie and Karen have spent a lot of time and energy researching this topic and attempting to relay it in an understandable form. They also share my style of humor, so this will not be your typical, dry factoid – "here's my story" – type of publication. As I'm truly just a humble surgeon from Grand Rapids, I'll let Julie and Karen take over now for the necessary, but boring credentials section.

Thank you Dr. Baker. Let's hear it for a truly caring guy who understands that overweight people are people too. Yeahhhh !!!!! All right, simmer down now. On to the credentials section:

As you read previously, Dr. Baker specializes in bariatric surgery and has had significant experience as a general surgeon prior to his bariatric practice. He is board certified by the American Board of Surgery and is a Fellow of the American College of Surgery. He completed a Fellowship in Critical Care and holds an additional certificate for Critical Care through the American Board of Surgery. Dr. Baker presently serves as the Medical Director of the Surgical Intensive Care Units at Spectrum Hospital, and is an Assistant Professor of Surgery at Michigan State University. He is a member of the American Society for Bariatric Surgery, the American Medical Association, and the Society of Critical Care Medicine.

Dr. Baker is also a 2005 award nominee for the Outstanding Achievement Award of the American Society for Bariatric Surgery Foundation. This award is given for significant contributions to the advancement of bariatric surgery, and representation of the highest ideals of the ASBS. As a nominee for this award Dr. Baker stands alongside some of the greatest medical minds in the world today, and his innovative ideas and contributions are most worthy of the praise. He is also a proud past recipient of the American College of Surgeons Transplantation Award.

Dr. Baker has researched, published, and lectured extensively on the topics of morbid obesity, bariatric surgery, and surgical critical care, and is on the Editorial Board of the prestigious *Obesity Surgery* journal, a publication of international reputation in the medical community. He also helped develop a bio-absorbable staple line product to decrease bleeding and leaks from staple lines.[1] This product won the 2002 American Medical Innovation of the Year award.

Following the development of that sealant, Drs. Baker, Foote, and Kemmeter presented and published a landmark study on "*The Science of Stapling and Leaks*" in the *Obesity Surgery* journal.[2] Portions of this research were presented at the International Federation for the Surgery of Obesity (IFSO) Conference in Spain in 2003. The research received the prestigious international INAMED Award, which consisted of a 60 lb statue that had to be carted back to the USA and through customs in an unruly, coarse, wooden box.

The credentials that he considers most important though, are those of husband and father of nine (yes... **9**...) wonderful children! (No, he is not Catholic or Mormon, which are the most common questions he and his wife are asked when out in public.) He is a caring and attentive family man, and has even been known to take the afternoon off work to take all of his children to see a Harry Potter movie. He's even cut meetings short with us to make sure he made it to one of his kid's basketball games (and that's one of the few good reasons to cut short a meeting with us, we'll tell you!)

In addition to all his amazing credentials, he is actually a caring doctor with a wonderful bedside manner! It helps to have a doctor with a good sense of humor, but he's also very careful not to make you laugh right after surgery. Dr. Baker is also just an all around nice person who cares deeply about his patients, attempting to help them find new, healthy, and enjoyable lives. He and his partners have surrounded themselves with staff of a similar ethic, those who have intense empathy for their patients through the "thick and thin" of the whole weight loss process.

We truly believe that there are many other "Dr. Baker" type bariatric surgeons out there just ready, willing, and able to help you make this important decision, and carry you through to a happy ending if you choose to proceed. We've talked to many people across the country who've had positive experiences similar to ours, and we hope you find your "Dr. Baker" soon.

Unfortunately, however, we've talked to more people who've not found a "Dr. Baker," but instead have found a "Dr. Frankenstein," or worse, a "Dr. Jekyll and Mr. Hyde." It is for them that this book came into being. We hope you'll love yourself enough to expect that your doctor will care about you the way Dr. Baker and his partners care about their patients. You deserve nothing less.

SCOTT H. GLASS, M.S., M.A., LLP

Scott, Scott, Scott. What to say about Scott? We just love him!! Scott is a limited licensure psychologist in Dr. Baker's practice. He holds a Master degree in Counseling Psychology from Western Michigan University, and a Master degree in Exercise Physiology from the University of Michigan. Scott received his dual Bachelor degrees from Calvin College in Grand Rapids in the areas of Physical Education, and Recreation. He has also studied Rehabilitation Psychology at Michigan State University. (Yes folks, he's yet another overachiever in the bunch. He's attended almost as many education institutions as I have!)

Scott worked as an exercise physiologist for about six years, and then moved into the counseling arena, where he has since focused the majority of his time. In working with weight loss surgery patients, he now uses both disciplines for which he was educated and trained. He is a wonderful, caring man, with a peace about him that is comforting when times are tough. Scott is able to help patients through many of their emotional, physical, behavioral, and even spiritual struggles, and we know that we couldn't have done it without him.

Scott grew up with four brothers, so we've adopted him into our families so he'd finally have some sisters. Too bad he got stuck with us!! Better luck next time, buddy!

Scott tells us that his professional goal is to improve the health, productivity, and quality of life of his patients through effective counseling and leadership. We can swear under oath (and I don't take that lightly), that he meets and exceeds his goal each and every day.

CARRIE A. LIEBROCK, R.D.

Carrie Liebrock needs your help! She is a registered dietitian with the most unrealistic, pathetic, plastic food models you've ever seen in your life sitting on her desk! We know they're there to give patients ideas and show portion sizes, but she really needs new plastic food that looks even remotely real! For crying out loud, little kids have more realistic plastic food than Carrie has! Send your pledges to 1-900-HELP-CARRIE-NOW (just kidding).

We tease her about her silly plastic food every time we go in her office. I even had to tease her through the tears when I had stricture difficulties and couldn't eat anything. That's how bad the plastic food is; it makes you comment even when you're being self-absorbed. Maybe that was her evil plan all along...?

Anyway, Carrie is a serious ray of sunshine at Dr. Baker's practice, goofy plastic food or not. She received her Bachelor of Science degree in Dietetics from the College of Human Ecology at Michigan State University. Two years later, Carrie completed a Dietetic Internship Certification in South Dakota, and presently serves as a registered dietitian at the MMPC® Center for Health Excellence.

Carrie has worked in several hospitals including Foote Hospital in Jackson, Michigan, Avera Sacred Heart Hospital in Yankton, South Dakota, and Covenant Health Care in Saginaw, Michigan. She's a wonderful source for nutrition information and practical weight loss strategies, and a delight to have around. We're very happy to be working with her on this project. We promise, in the interest of her patients, some of the proceeds from this book will go to buy her new plastic food

So now that we've introduced you to everyone, I bet you're wondering just how this book came to be. (Well, if you weren't we're going to tell you anyway.) It really wasn't because Dr. Baker asked us to write one. By the time he met us, he'd pretty much stopped asking patients to write a book because no one seemed to have either the time, or the inclination. Nope. This book came about in a whole different way. Here's the real skinny on the...

BIRTH OF A BOOK

The inspiration for this book came from a rather strange source: a garage sale. In the summer of 2004, Karen and I found ourselves gasping for air under a mountain of "too big" clothes. We'd already shrunk through about four sizes each when we decided to have a garage sale and let others adopt our beloved clothing. After all, many of them were never worn, and some still even had the tags attached. As each piece was lovingly hunted down in true bargain-hunter style, we simply couldn't let them rot and mold in a garage somewhere, so we put them up for sale.

As professional women, we both have to dress up for work, and the money we'd put into our clothes was significant. A garage sale was our only hope of recouping some of the cash (we needed new clothes...), and seeing our beloved treasures go to good and loving homes. Lots of people came to the sale (more for the man junk my husband had out there than for the clothes), but soon a trend began to emerge.

The majority of the women who were there to look at the clothes also had weight loss surgery. Of course, they were curious as to why two women were selling a Bloomingdale's worth of clothing, and in no time at all a bond was forming over scars, clothes, tears, and lost pounds.

What struck us though, were the stories that accompanied those scars. You see, Karen and I have virtually no scars to speak of, while *all* of the women we met had great long scars up their torsos from their surgeries. They told stories of how they got those scars too, and all of them involved a mass of miscommunications, omissions, and outdated information.

The stories centered around women (and they told of men they knew as well), that were sick of their weight issues and sought knowledge and help from medical professionals they trusted, literally, with their lives. We heard story after story of people who went to this center, and that clinic, and received not much more service than you get from the overworked and underpaid waitress at a greasy spoon.

We heard stories like the one told to us by a young woman who went to a bariatric surgery clinic, was told briefly about the surgery, and waited while they checked to see if her insurance would pay. They sent her home to wait for an authorization, and when it was received they booked her surgery. She showed up at the hospital on surgery day, had a full open procedure done ("zippers" I call them), spent one and a half days in the hospital, and was sent home. She was told to drink Slimfast®, and to come back to the office in two weeks to have her stitches out.

When she showed up two weeks later, they removed her stitches, handed her a meal plan on a single sheet of paper, and wished her well. No orientation, no pre-operative testing, no counseling, no follow-up, no nutritional counseling, no answers to her questions – nothing. Just thanks for the money and the memories lady. See ya, wouldn't want to be ya.

By the way, our young friend was experiencing horrible nausea and diarrhea multiple times a day. She had the shakes, and would break out in cold sweats. She said she was worried she had a heart problem because her heart would race so. When she called for help in dealing with these symptoms, her surgeon's office said it wasn't his area, and to call her primary care physician.

She was stunned when we told her that the large quantity of orange and apple juice she was taking in six to seven times a day was probably what was making her sick; a phenomenon known as dumping syndrome (see Chapter Five entitled "Auto Eject"). Since two weeks after her surgery, her surgeon's office recommended she drink fruit juices all day long to curb her need to eat sweets and other foods. Apparently no one told her that too much sugar would make her sick, not to mention she was ingesting tons of calories that weren't giving her much nutrition, giving her no protein, and not helping her feel full or satisfied.

We also heard from a 5 foot 10 inch woman who only (it's all relative...) had ninety pounds to lose, who also had a zipper-procedure done. She was in tears when she saw (or rather had to help hunt for), Karen's almost non-existent laparoscopic incision scars. We were appalled at the assembly line approach that was taken in her case as well. Again, no orientation, no counseling, no medical work-up, no follow-up. Nothing. Just here's your bill, and don't let the operating room door hit you in the butt on the way out!

When we told these people of our experiences with weight loss surgery, there were more than a few tears of envy and regret I'll tell you. We reasoned there simply had to be a place to go for people who need potentially life-saving information in order to get the real scoop and skinny from people who've been there, not just people who stand to make a profit from others' misery. Thus, this book was born.

Karen and I talked it over, and because we're two college professors whose job it is to research, write, and bring the light of knowledge to the masses (pathetic, isn't it...), we decided that we were the perfect people to write this book; except for the medical part.

For that we needed Dr. Baker: our friend, our physician, our trusted medical savior. So we cornered him at the hospital on the way into surgery, and told him he was going to co-author a book to help people just like the patient lying there on the gurney before him. Not exactly in a position to say no, he agreed, and we had witnesses.

Actually, we did corner him at the hospital, but he was more than exhilarated to be a part of this project. He was all pumped up about it, and had thoughts and ideas just flying through his mind. He was virtually bouncing around the room with excitement as he left to go back to surgery. I often wonder about that day... and, well... I hope things went okay for that patient, and the surgery wasn't too delicate a procedure. I've never asked, but I'm sure all went just swimmingly....

So, here it is. The culmination of a lot of thinking, sharing, analysis, research, experience, and caring. We all hope that you find the answers and the information you need in this book. If nothing else, at least find the questions you need to ask to save your own life.

In the immortal (paraphrased) words
from Shakespeare's Macbeth, "Read on, Macduff."

Don't be afraid

that your life will end...

be afraid that

it will never begin.

GRACE HANSON

Chapter Three

THE NEW AND IMPROVED, AMAZING ALL NATURAL LEMON DIET

Randal S. Baker, M.D., F.A.C.S.

…Stay tuned for scenes from tomorrow's episode of <u>As The Stomach Turns</u>. And now a word from our sponsor:

(Announcer) Are you tired of struggling with your weight? Tired of all the typical diets without any success? Is the mirror considered one of your foes? Do you need more energy, and want to break free from the heavy bondage of extra weight? Does your sex life need help? Is climbing stairs a chore? Sick of the décor at Subway®? High blood pressure getting you down? Is fat around your belly, hips, and thighs a source of entertainment at family gatherings? Well the answer is finally here! Doc Baker's New and Improved, Amazing, All Natural Lemon Diet.

Yes, you heard right. Nature has provided the necessary weight combating "delta force" in this lemon-based anti-fat, anti-oxidant, low-carb, low-sugar, anti-leptin, anti-ghrelin, appetite-suppressing, sleep-improving, non-stimulant, caffeine-free, ephedra-free, recipe-enhancing dietary supplement. One pinch of this potent concentrated lemon extract before each meal and every mouthful of food will just chase the calories away.

Why, Hanky Snider of Hooterville, Arkansas, lost 40 pounds in just one month using Doc's powerful and amazing, all natural lemon-based elixir. Hanky, who once shunned being seen in public, now leads tours through extensive subterranean caves. "Many of my tour people have asked the secret of my youthful vitality, energy, and weight loss. I tell them they must check out Doc's health-inducing, all natural, cortisol-blocking, age-reversing, skin-tightening, intestinal-cleansing, fat-trapping, hair-growing supplement. It's the greatest!"

Even model-actress Barbie Beauty lost 30 pounds in only two weeks using the life-enhancing, strength-reviving product. "Why, I even lost weight while sleeping at night, and dropped 3 dress sizes to a 2. And I wasn't even dreaming about weight loss or exercise! Huh… Anyway, all the studios are calling now, and I've had to hire a secretary just to answer my calls! Thanks, Doc Baker. You're my hero!"

Sound unbelievable? Well it is!!! Doc Baker's New and Improved, Amazing, All Natural Lemon Diet is much too powerful for those of you *who only have a couple of vanity pounds to lose. Noooo! You need to be seriously stretched out of shape, at least triple your high school gradua-tion weight, and dissolving from the inside out to be using Doc's Diet. And because we know you no longer want to be mistaken for a float in the Macy's Thanksgiving Day parade, we're only charging $169.99 a bottle for Doc's miracle diet compound. And, if you call now, we'll even send you a second bottle **free** because we know you really need the help. That's TWO bottles of Doc's lemon miracle for only $169.99, plus $10.00 shipping and handling.*

Just try it for yourself! Find out what millions of other grateful and satisfied customers have discovered. They're sold on Doc Baker's New and Improved, Amazing, All Natural Lemon Diet, and you will be too! There's a 100% money back guarantee if you're not totally satisfied! (Just return the bottle with original proof of purchase and the kneecaps of two West African newts and we will completely refund your money!)

What are you waiting for? Call now! 1-999-BIG-CURE. That's 1-999-BIG-CURE. Again, that's 1-999-BIG-CURE. Operators are standing by! Why be fat, ugly, and disease-ridden when you can miraculously change all that, guaranteed? Make the choice for a healthy and a leaner, more beautiful and vivacious body! Buy Doc's all natural, cortisol-binding, weight loss inducing, life-rejuvenating, lemon-based supplement! Call today!

(Results depicted are not typical. Individual results may vary.)

Does this diet diatribe sound all too familiar? A hundred years ago, "snake oil" salesmen used the same pitch to sell their tonics that were guaranteed to "cure what-ever ailed ya!" Today, the weight loss "snake oil" salesmen abound, and money spent on diets and weight related products are in the billions. Just slap up some before and after pictures of non-typical customers along with some medical sounding jargon, and almost anything sells as the new version of "snake oil." An overweight, stressed-out, desperate America is looking to any and every "snake oil" salesman for help and a cure for its obesity and weight related problems.

Although we all use the terms "obese," and "overweight" interchangeably in con-versation, medical definitions of the condition exist — and yes, obesity is considered a real health "condition." The National Institutes of Health (NIH) states that a person is considered "obese" when he or she weighs 20 percent or more than his or her ideal body weight. At this point, the person's weight poses a real health risk. Obesity be-comes "morbid" when it *significantly* increases the risk of one or more obesity-related health conditions or serious diseases.

According to national and international researchers, statistics now show that 65% of the U.S. population are overweight or obese, approximately six percent of Americans are morbidly obese, and nearly half a billion of the world's population is now considered overweight or obese.[1] Morbid obesity is a serious chronic disease, meaning that its symptoms build slowly over an extended period of time. The media inundates us with images of "perfect" bodies from childhood on, and yet the obesity epidemic is one of the fastest growing diseases ever! In response, people are always searching for the "easy" way out, the "magic pill," or the "silver bullet;" the instant, simple, no effort required, quick fix for being overweight.

This then, begs the question of what causes obesity. Why is obesity dramatically increasing in our society? Like so many ailments such as alcoholism, the cause is directly related to genetics and environment.[2] Many alcoholics have a genetic predisposition towards alcoholism in that drinking alcohol stimulates certain portions of their brain more so than non-alcoholics.[3]

In obesity, we see that many family relatives share the predisposition toward being overweight. In fact, identical twins separated from birth will both usually have similar weights (including obesity), despite different environmental backgrounds.[4]

Environmental concerns are also important. Overall, obesity is rising as we change our environment from that of our predecessors. We no longer have to run on foot to hunt for food, or labor physically to plant and harvest crops. We do not have to work to prepare and store food either. Food is readily available, especially in calorie dense forms, and is sold in "bigger" sizes. Portion sizes have increased dramatically over the past years as well, and our "bigger" sizes today would have been considered mega-gargantuan in the previous century.

The "typical" 20th century American arises after too little sleep, and eats a breakfast of chocolate super-frosted-sugar balls, while working hard to "hunt" for, and click on the remote to the television. They then "run" to the car, and scurry off to "work" which for many consists of an exhausting day behind a desk typing on a computer. Break time is really more of the same, including sitting and eating snack cakes, soda pop, and way too much coffee. Lunch often consists of "flying" to a fast food restaurant, and not having the gumption to refuse the obnoxious siren call to "super size" your already "bigger sized," calorie packed meal.

Today, in large part, our created environments have allowed genetic predispositions to become dominant and rampant. Poor diets and lack of exercise have even lead to obesity in people who do not have clear familial genetic predispositions.[5] According to the Surgeon General, we are as a nation, dying at varying rates from obesity.[6]

Health care professionals often fail to recognize these multifactorial genetic and environmental predispositions associated with obesity. They sometimes label patients as lazy, unmotivated, or lacking will power. Although that may occasionally be the case, these descriptors are not generally major factors in a vast majority of patient obesity conditions.[7]

As I have given lectures around the country on obesity and obesity surgery, I have confronted intense biases toward obese people. Obesity prejudice is one of the last few remaining bastions of politically correct snobbery. Studies reveal that obese people are prejudged by the general public to be lazy, stupid, unorganized, selfish, and inept.[8] When faced with two substitute teachers who did identical teaching, even school children judged the skinny sub to be the best teacher in all respects.[9] This response is simply an outcropping of a greater societal prejudice that has developed regarding overweight people – a term I call "obesism."

Obesism has infiltrated the medical community despite the intellectual knowledge that obesity is a disease. As a result, obese patients are handed prescriptions that say, "lose weight," or are given poor quality, one-sheet "diet plans," and expected to lose weight. It is like handing a long time drug addict a script that says, "Stop taking drugs." I've even heard one physician tout his well thought out, overarching, anti-obesity plan by announcing in the hospital ward "send them all to the 'fat' farm." What insight….

So, we're living in a society that is biased against overweight people, and face it, you're probably biased too. Even overweight people view other overweight people with such a bias. If we all look at overweight people with such disdain, and we can't resolve that bias even knowing it's false, then the only thing left to do is to resolve the underlying cause. Let's treat the obesity itself, without adding in any obesism biases.

In order to do that, we must base our plan on **evidence,** not just hearsay based on rumor and conjecture sprinkled liberally with personal, non-evidence-oriented gestalt (unless of course you prefer "snake oil" to scientifically based research). In this case, the evidence is overwhelming! In examining the evidence, let's start with a uniform definition and standard for the terms *overweight, obese*, and *morbidly obese.*

In order to consistently describe and properly treat obesity, a uniform medical standard is used. This is called the Body Mass Index (BMI). The BMI takes into account weight and height, but not age, gender, frame size, or muscle mass which vary significantly from patient to patient. Because these variables are so far ranging, the only way to standardize obesity is to use the two factors that can be consistently compared – height and weight. When considering a person's BMI, a 5 feet tall, 300 pound person is considered to be in worse medical straits than a 7 feet tall, 300 pound person, no matter their age, gender, frame size, or muscle mass.

Persons considered to be *normal weight,* have a BMI under 25. Any BMI over 25 is considered to be in the *overweight* category. *Obese* refers to a BMI of 30-39. *Morbid obesity,* sometimes called *"clinically severe obesity,"* is defined as being 100 pounds or more over ideal body weight, or having a BMI of greater than 40.

For the overweight, obese, and morbidly obese, temporary weight loss is not the solution. Temporarily losing weight, gaining it back, and then losing weight again is what we term "yo-yo" dieting. Yo-yo dieting has been shown to be detrimental to your health.[10] True weight loss success must be measured in loss of extra weight over **years** not months.

Almost every "diet miracle" in the media emphasizes the short term, initial weight loss. "I lost ten pounds in just seven days on the incredible green paint diet." So, maybe you lost ten pounds in seven days, but how did you lose it? Did you keep it off? For how long? Did you lose any more? Did you die from the stupid green paint?

The true test of a diet program's success is to see where participants settle in 3-5 years. Studies have shown that long-term loss of only 10-15% of excess body weight significantly improves many weight related medical problems.[11] For morbidly obese patients the data also unfortunately shows that there is a less than 2% long-term success rate for even the best medically supervised weight loss programs![12] In most studies that look at sustained weight loss for longer than 3 years, the number is closer to zero![13]

Now suppose that you were told by your physician that you had a medical condition that significantly decreased your longevity (life span), carried a significantly increased risk for multiple cancers, was associated with multiple medical problems that would require a myriad of medications, and would adversely affect virtually every organ in your body. Your doctor then wrote you out a prescription and said, "Here, take this. It usually works around 0% of the time long term."

Unfortunately, most general health care professionals treat patients this way, acting as if their advice to lose weight and "diet" will have more than a modicum of a chance of success. In fact, most never track their patients' results to be able to report any reasonable or verifiable data on their treatment methods. I guess that leaves overweight patients standing out in the cold, with no way to solve their weight issues or the medically related problems. Enter: the surgical treatment option.

The NIH states that surgery for obesity is largely reserved for those approximately 100 pounds overweight, with a BMI of 40 or greater – the morbidly obese. The NIH established recommendations regarding weight loss surgery back in 1992, and the American Society of Bariatric Surgery and American Society for Bariatric Physicians defer to those recommendations as well. Basically, a patient who has failed previous attempts at weight loss, with a BMI of 40 or greater is a candidate. If you have tried medically supervised programs, even if you've lost weight on those programs, it will count toward meeting the criteria if you've put the weight back on.

The NIH recommendations did not, however, define a "supervised program." As practitioners, we interpret this to mean a significant attempt at weight loss under physician supervision. The best model is a totally supervised medical program where physicians are involved and monitor all aspects of the program. Also acceptable is the situation in which a primary care doctor monitors a patient while they under go such programs as Weight Watchers® or Jenny Craig®.

Patients who do not meet the NIH criteria because of a BMI that is too low, who are unable to stop smoking, have acute mental illness, are current substance abusers (including alcohol), have had a Myocardial Infarction (M.I.) or stroke within the previous six months, or are less than five years out from treatment for certain types of cancers, are *not*, in our view, candidates for weight loss surgery.

Having a BMI over 40, however, is not the only criterion for weight loss surgery. Just having a BMI over 25 can lead to multiple related medical problems, referred to as co-morbidities. Those with high-risk, co-morbid conditions, and a BMI of between 35 and 40 also meet the NIH criteria for surgery. Weight related co-morbidities include type II diabetes, high blood pressure (hypertension), stroke, coronary artery disease (CAD), obstructive sleep apnea (OSA), congestive heart failure (CHF), hypoventilation syndrome, gallbladder disease, hyperlipidemia (high cholesterol), headaches, gastro-esophageal acid reflux (heartburn), degenerative joint disease, polycystic ovary syndrome, infertility, menstrual irregularities, endometrial cancer, breast cancer, prostate cancer, colon cancer, osteoarthritis (OA), cardiac and respiratory dysfunction, gout, depression, Alzheimer's, premature death, deep vein thrombosis (DVT), pulmonary emboli (blood clot to lungs), stress urinary incontinence, and others.

All of these conditions can occur in the absence of obesity, but all are significantly increased when obesity is present. In time, most morbidly obese patients will develop a good number of these medical problems, often requiring multiple medications and occasionally surgery to control the maladies, and resulting in a decreased quality of life.[14]

Additionally, obesity related costs greatly affect our country's economy when you figure in the cost of medications for all of the above mentioned medical problems, and the loss of worker productivity from obesity related sickness and leave.[15] Many younger people with morbid obesity are also on disability for obesity related conditions.[16] Finally, there is the staggering amount of hard-earned, and for many, hard-come-by dollars spent on diets and weight related-drugs and programs that simply have no hope of having any real effect.

So, why consider such a "radical" approach to obesity if it is basically caused by a series of unfortunate genes, and a lifetime of "poor" lifestyle choices? The simple answer: to help patients *live*.

The quality of life issues related to obesity are numerous and significant. Many of my morbidly obese patients often cannot sit in normal chairs or seats, perform basic hygiene, clip their own nails, work, help others in physically related tasks, or even breathe without assistance. These people may believe they have received a rotten hand in the big deal of life, and maybe they didn't play their cards well on top of it, but they deserve the same chance for a happy, healthy, productive life as anyone else. (Anyone who thinks otherwise needs a serious bias and attitude adjustment.)

Helping people find that better life is why we consider such "radical" treatments as surgical intervention. You know, that "radical-high-risk-experimental surgery that didn't work on my wife's second cousin's aunt, twice removed? Well, this ain't your wife's second cousin's aunt, twice removed's old fashioned stomach stapling procedure anymore!

Surgical approaches to the treatment of obesity came as a result of the lack of efficacy of medical weight loss programs, and the significant adverse effects associated with morbid obesity. As I give a very basic overview of the history of weight loss surgery, it may help you to refer to the illustration of the gastrointestinal tract on the next page, and the glossary we provided in the back of the book, or on the web site if the illustrations and explanations are not sufficient.

©2005

FIGURE 3.1 — Gastrointestinal Tracts

1. The esophagus is a long muscular tube, which moves food from the mouth to the stomach.

2. The abdomen contains all of the digestive organs.

3. The stomach, situated at the top of the abdomen, normally holds just over 3 pints (about 1500 ml) of food from a single meal. Here the food is mixed with an acid that is produced to assist in digestion. In the stomach, acid and other digestive juices are added to the ingested food to facilitate breakdown of complex proteins, fats and carbohydrates into small, more absorbable units.

4. A valve at the entrance to the stomach from the esophagus allows the food to enter while keeping the acid-laden food from "refluxing" back into the esophagus, causing damage and pain.

5. The pylorus is a small round muscle located at the outlet of the stomach and the entrance to the duodenum (the first section of the small intestine). It closes the stomach outlet while food is being digested into a smaller, more easily absorbed form. When food is properly digested, the pylorus opens and allows the contents of the stomach into the duodenum.

6. The small intestine is about 15 to 20 feet long (4.5 to 6 meters) and is where the majority of the absorption of the nutrients from food takes place. The small intestine is made up of three sections: the duodenum, the jejunum and the ileum.

7. The duodenum is the first section of the small intestine and is where the food is mixed with bile produced by the liver and with other juices from the pancreas. This is where much of the iron and calcium is absorbed.

8. The jejunum is the middle part of the small intestine extending from the duodenum to the ileum; it is responsible for digestion.

9. The last segment of the intestine, the ileum, is where the absorption of fat-soluble vitamins A, D, E and K and other nutrients are absorbed.

10. Another valve separates the small and large intestines to keep bacteria-laden colon contents from coming back into the small intestine.

11. In the large intestines, excess fluids are absorbed and a firm stool is formed. The colon may absorb protein, when necessary.

(information courtesy of Ethicon Endo-Surgery, Inc.)

Surgical weight loss treatment can be done two ways. The first is described as a "malabsorptive" technique which means that many of the calories consumed are not absorbed, and pass through the system. The second is a "restrictive" technique meaning a small pouch is created out of the stomach to give the feeling of fullness from much less food. A third option was developed combining the malabsorptive and restrictive techniques.

In the 70's the most popular surgical approach was called the *jejuno-ileal* or *intestinal bypass,* and it was purely malabsorptive. In this surgery the majority of the small bowel (where nutrients are absorbed) was bypassed by hooking up the small bowel in a different way. This procedure was easy to perform, and at first seemed to have good weight loss. The problem with this approach is that people developed severe diarrhea from the malabsorption.

In addition, many electrolytes (sodium and potassium, for example) were adversely affected and hospitalization for replacement of these electrolytes was not infrequent. Many patients developed severe protein depletion, as they could not adequately absorb protein, and this many times required an I.V. and TPN (liquid food via vein). Finally, the bypassed portion of small bowel grew bacteria that adversely affected the liver, sometimes leading to liver failure. As a result, this procedure was abandoned.

©2005

FIGURE 3.2 — Jejuno-ileal Bypass End to End

©2005

FIGURE 3.3 — Jejuno-ileal Bypass End to Side

There are three main, purely "restrictive" types of weight loss surgeries. One is called a *gastroplasty*, where the stomach is simply stapled to form a smaller pouch, but the small intestine is left intact. The second is called a *vertical banded gastroplasty* (VBG) during which a hole is stapled in the center of the stomach, a vertical line is stapled from the top of the hole to the upper edge of the stomach, and a vertical band is attached from the side of the hole to the edge of the stomach in order to restrict food intake. The third is called an Adjustable Gastric Banding procedure, and I'll talk more about that later in the chapter.

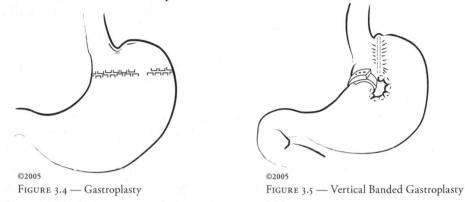

©2005
FIGURE 3.4 — Gastroplasty

©2005
FIGURE 3.5 — Vertical Banded Gastroplasty

With the development of a new technique, the *biliopancreatic diversion,* came one variant of the combination of the restrictive and malabsorptive techniques. This procedure was an improvement on the jejuno-ileal bypass in that no small intestine lost function, thereby decreasing damage to the liver. Biliopancreatic diversion patients tend to suffer from protein deficiency, stomach ulcers, diarrhea, and foul smelling flatulence. A modified version of this procedure, called the *duodenal switch,* is still done today, but more so in Europe and other countries than in the U.S. In general, these procedures tend to have better overall weight loss, but at the expense of increased complications, and are not very popular in North America.

©2005
FIGURE 3.6 — Biliopancreatic Diversion

©2005
FIGURE 3.7 — Biliopancreatic Diversion with Duodenal Switch

The *Roux-en-Y gastric bypass (RYGB),* which is both malabsorptive and restrictive, was originally created in the 1960s and involves using medical staplers to create a small pouch in the top part of the stomach. To give you a good mental visual, the pouch is generally not any bigger than an egg. The rest of the stomach is not removed, but is stapled shut on top, and remains connected to the small bowel below. Bile from the gallbladder and pancreatic juices are released through the remainder portion of the stomach, and into the small bowel. The remainder portion of the stomach still creates stomach acids as well. These acids are necessary for the breakdown of foods in the gastrointestinal tract.

The small bowel then carries these digestive acids downstream where they meet with the food coming in through the new small pouch, aiding in nutrient absorption. A piece of the small bowel is then brought up to the new pouch to allow empty-ing of food contents directly into the bowel (the "Roux" limb). The procedure also constructs a tiny stomach outlet, which slows the speed food leaves your new "egg" stomach. Satiety (a feeling of fullness), is created when the pouch is filled with small amounts of food that tells the brain the walls of the stomach are stretched and full.

A very small malabsorptive component is present from the bypass of some small bowel used to create the "Y" of the Roux-en-Y configuration. Several variants of the Roux-en-Y surgery exist, and if you choose to have a Roux-en-Y surgery, you should be clear which procedure your surgeon will use.

Incidentally, the name "Roux" comes from the surgeon who first divided, and reconnected the small bowel in a similar pattern, and the "Y" comes from the shape or route the bowel then takes after surgery; it looks like a capital "Y." (At least it looks like a "Y" to surgeons. Don't feel bad if you can't really see it. It's one of those "you have to be there" things.)

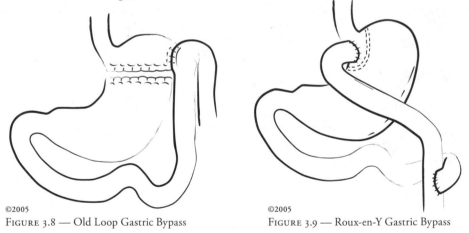

©2005   ©2005
FIGURE 3.8 — Old Loop Gastric Bypass   FIGURE 3.9 — Roux-en-Y Gastric Bypass

According to many weight loss experts, the RYGB is considered to be the "gold standard" for surgical weight loss procedures as it has a good, long-term track re-cord.[17] It can be done by creating a full abdominal incision (an "open" procedure) in order to lift the liver out of the way, and access the stomach and small intestine, but the need to use this particular method has drastically decreased in recent years with the move toward laparoscopic methods.

Open procedure incisions for women tend to be about 4 ½ to 6 inches long, and about 5 ½ to 7 inches for men. The RYGB can now be done via a laparoscope (camera placed into the body through small incisions). Six small incisions are made in the abdomen into which instrument portals and the laparoscope are inserted. The procedure is now performed laparoscopically more often than by open incision in the U.S.

©2005

FIGURE 3.10 — Placement of Open Incision

©2005

FIGURE 3.11 — Placement of Laparoscopic Incisions

RYGB patients can plan to spend 3-4 days in the hospital if an "open" procedure is required. At our center, in approximately 97% of cases, my partners and I are able to perform the procedure laparoscopically, and the hospital stay is then generally 1-2 days. Patients often go back to work in 1-2 weeks following laparoscopic surgery, or 4-6 weeks after an open procedure, especially if their work involves activity such as bending or lifting.

Patients are on a liquid protein diet for approximately two weeks before surgery in order to shrink the liver, and clear the intestinal tract of food substances. The liver must be shrunk to its smallest size possible as it sits directly in front of the stomach, and must be lifted by instruments and held out of the way. Some livers are very heavy, and if the liver can't be lifted out of the way with the laparoscopic instruments, the surgery may have to be converted to an open procedure involving a much bigger incision.

Shrinking the liver through use of the liquid protein diet helps the patient's chances of having a laparoscopic procedure, and with every pound gone prior to surgery, the patient's chances of cardiac and respiratory complications decrease. Patients then continue on a liquid protein diet for approximately two weeks following surgery (protocols may vary slightly from surgeon to surgeon and patient to patient), while the stomach and small intestine heal.

Patients usually graduate to soft foods as tolerated at around two weeks post surgery. After four weeks have passed, patients may then begin eating more solid foods as tolerated. Many RYGB patients experience an intolerance of certain foods for a while, something that Julie and Karen will discuss further in the next chapter.

The advantage of the laparoscopic RYGB approach includes a decreased risk of wound infections and hernias, decreased pain, decreased length of hospital stay, and decreased post-operative restrictions. The laparoscopic approach also produces fewer adhesions (scars) on the inside of the abdomen. This means that in the future, if other unrelated surgeries are needed, there will be fewer adhesions to potentially complicate the procedure.

As with all surgeries, however, complications can develop. Leaks, strictures, bleeding, infections, pulmonary emboli, and other complications can occur. Complications from Roux-en-Y surgery will be discussed a little later in this chapter.

Overall, nationally reported mortality (death) rates from Roux-en-Y surgery are around .5%, which is less than more malabsorptive procedures, but more than purely restrictive procedures.[18] At our center the mortality rate is less than .2% for RYGB. Deaths most often occur from pulmonary emboli that are blood clots that form in the legs and pass to the lung, blocking blood flow.[19]

A variant of the RYGB procedure now being done is often called the *"mini-Roux-en-Y."* The stomach is still stapled into a small, albeit usually longer pouch, but the small bowel is not separated to bring up a Roux limb. Instead the small bowel is connected to the pouch in a loop fashion. The procedure takes somewhat less time, but can significantly increase the risk of ulceration from bile and acid refluxing up to the pouch as the loop allows these substances easier access to the pouch. Bile and acid reflux into the pouch can be painful, and may increase the risk of cancer developing.[20] Based on this data, many bariatric surgeons frown upon this type of bypass.

©2005

FIGURE 3.12 — Mini Gastric Bypass

Another recent addition to the bariatric surgery field is the laparoscopic *Adjustable Gastric Band* (commonly referred to as a Lap-Band®). This technique involves placing an adjustable silicone band around the top of the stomach to create a small pouch. This balloon type band is connected to a port, which goes under the skin so the surgeon can inject saline solution into the band to expand it, and thus adjust the band and the size of the food "pouch" created.

Note, I said the surgeon can adjust the band, as a patient has been known to attempt to deflate the band by himself before a vacation cruise. Unfortunately, the patient kept the saline from the band in an unsterile container during the food fest, and then attempted to re-inject the now infected fluid back in the port. A nasty infection then followed, requiring removal of the band.

Normally, the band and food cause distension (expansion) of the small pouch, and thus satiety. This procedure does not involve stapling the stomach or bowel, and is therefore somewhat less invasive. It is adjustable and reversible, two benefits not associated with RYGB. The down side is that patients tend to lose weight more slowly than with the RYGB, and overall in most cases lose less weight as compared to RYGB patients.[21]

©2005
FIGURE 3.13 — Adjustable Gastric Band (Lap-Band®)

In our experience the Lap-Band® should be considered for patients who cannot have an RYGB because they may have: Crohn's Disease, have had other lower abdominal surgeries that do not facilitate an RYGB procedure, have certain medical conditions such as Irritable Bowel Syndrome (IBS) or Celiac Disease, are less than five years from a malignancy, or are very high risk patients that may not survive the restructuring of their stomach and gastrointestinal tract. Patients who are at the lower end of the morbid obesity scale may also be ideal patients.

It takes approximately one hour to perform this surgery, and patients are commonly in the hospital overnight. Patients usually return to work in 1 to 2 weeks, but must generally be evaluated every 6 to 8 weeks for gradual adjustment of the band.

Patients report having good weight loss with the Lap-Band® (approximately 1-2 pounds per week). They complain of difficulty eating thick meats and breads, and like RYGB patients they must cut their food into small bites, and chew it extremely well. Also like RYGB patients, Lap-Band® patients should not drink liquids with meals, nor consume calories solely in liquid form (juice, protein drinks, milk shakes).

The Lap-Band® patient is generally on clear liquids for the first two days, transitioning to soft foods for 2-4 weeks, and then to solid foods at the fourth week. Although most studies also show better weight loss with the RYGB, Lap-Band® patients who are very compliant with their weight loss program can have results that match the RYGB. (Unless one tries to self-adjust the band!)

There are always risks with any surgery. Surgical complications can't always be prevented, but the risks can be minimized. You and your doctor must weigh any potential complications against the risks of not having the procedure at all. The potential complications of bariatric surgery include, but are not limited to:

Stricture: *Stenosis*, or narrowing of the connection between the stomach pouch and intestine that may require a procedure to correct the narrowing. Stricture is the most common type of complication seen with RYGB, occurring statistically in 5-8% of patients. Lap-Band® patients can experience a version of this complication if the band is too tight around the top of the stomach. Most patients notice difficulty with tolerating solids and if the opening is very tight even taking in liquids will be difficult. Nausea and vomiting can develop. Many patients describe reflux of white type "foam" and this usually indicates a tight stricture. Strictures tend to show up around three weeks after surgery and are treated by an endoscope placed down through the mouth into the pouch. A balloon is then used through the scope to dilate (stretch open) the tight area. Most patients only need this done one time, although occasionally strictures require several dilation sessions.

Gallstones: Historically, as many as 30% of patients were thought to develop gallstones after RYGB. This number is probably much lower and is related to the weight loss that occurs with bariatric procedures, rather than the bariatric procedure itself. Symptomatic gallstones are usually treated by removal of the gallbladder, which can most times be performed laparoscopically. The risk of gallstones can be decreased by the patient taking bile salts for six months after surgery, however this approach is very expensive. In the past, many surgeons advocated always taking out the gallbladder at the time of bariatric surgery. Today, however, most surgeons use a selective approach by only removing the gallbladder if the patient has gall stones and/or has symptoms from gall stones. It is a whole lot easier to take a gallbladder out laparoscopically if the patient loses significant weight as the gallbladder is directly under the liver.

Bleeding during or after surgery: This complication is seen with virtually any type of surgery, and occurs in approximately 1-2% of bariatric surgical patients. It is sometimes treated with a blood infusion, or in the case of a persistent bleed, the patient may have to return to surgery to have the source of the bleeding stopped. Bleeding can occur from the staple lines, liver, spleen, and other organs or even from an incision. Often patients are given low doses of blood thinners (Heparin) to decrease the risk of blood clots. This can make patients more "oozy" around the time of surgery. Some bleeding though is far better than dealing with blood clots that could pass to the lungs. Use of staple buttressing material has been shown to decrease bleeding and may be helpful for decreasing this risk.

Pneumonia: As with any medical procedure that involves full anesthesia, patients can develop pneumonia, or fluid in the lungs. Pneumonia occurs statistically in less than 2% of all patients. This can often be prevented by getting the patient up and about as soon as possible, as well as by having the patient breath into a plastic device called a "spirometer" to help re-expand the lungs and prevent collapse. Patients who previously smoked or have sleep apnea and underlying lung disorders are at a higher risk for pneumonia.

Hernia: This is one of the more common complications seen in patients who have an open incision surgery. It occurs in up to 40 % of non-laparoscopic RYGB surgeries.

A hernia is a protrusion through an abnormal opening in the fascia layer of the abdomen that keeps the abdominal contents inside. Hernias require another operation to fix the problem, and can be complex and difficult to repair. Until much of the weight is off, the hernia can recur, as there is too much pressure on the belly, which reopens the hernia. This complication of open surgery is probably one of the most frustrating to many surgeons. It often involves reopening the edge of the hernia to find the fascia. There are usually a lot of adhesions around this area, and these must be taken down to free up the fascia all around so the hernia defect can be closed. Often some type of mesh is needed to give additional strength to the repair. Overall this complication represents one of the major reasons to consider a laparoscopic approach.

Leaks: Leaks can occur in the staple line or at the connections of the bowel to itself, or the stomach pouch. Leaks occur in approximately 2-3% of RYGB patients. Lap-Band® patients do not usually experience this complication, although a leak originating from where the band was placed on the stomach, and the bottom of the swallowing tube has been reported. Most leaks occur within 24-36 hours and present with abnormal vital signs (temperatures, heart rates) and elevated white cell counts. A contrast swallow study is sometimes performed to help with the diagnosis of a leak. Stronger staple lines and fewer leaks are associated with the use of staple line buttressing material. Leaks most often require additional surgery to attempt to close the leak, and drain the leak area in case the closure does not hold. The tissue around a leak can become weak and does not always hold sutures well so the drains assure the leak will remain "controlled" and eventually heal up over time.

Pulmonary embolus: Commonly referred to as a blood clot in the lung, it is a risk for all persons undergoing any type of surgery. The clots block blood flow in part of the lung and decrease the body's ability to get enough oxygen. Statistically, the risk for this complication in all RYGB surgery is less than 1% of patients. Preventative measures for this complication are mainly in avoiding clots forming in the legs through the use of blood thinning agents and other measures.

Deep vein thrombosis (DVT): DVT means a blood clot in the large veins of the leg. While in the legs, the blood clots are painful, but they become most serious when they float up into the blood vessels of the lungs, thereby becoming pulmonary emboli. Prevention methods include wearing compression stockings, taking blood thinners, and walking as soon as possible after surgery. People at high risk for clots may need to have a filter placed in the large vein in the abdomen that drains all the leg veins. This filter can decrease the risk of clots moving to the lungs where they become a pulmonary embolism.

Infections: Infections in the wound or abdomen can occur after any abdominal surgery. Wound infections are more common in open procedures and especially in patients who have diabetes and an open incision. Sometimes opening up the outer incision, and courses of antibiotics are needed to cure wound infections. Occasionally, a collection of infection in the abdomen (abscess) will need to be drained using CT scan directed drains.

Bowel obstruction: A partial or full blockage of the bowel can occur after abdominal surgery. Most of these blockages occur weeks to months out from surgery but can even occur years later. One cause for this is adhesions that can develop purely from the act of performing surgery in the abdomen. This is more common with open surgery, as the large incision causes more adhesions to form. Another type of blockage is from an internal hernia. Openings created to connect the small bowel together, or to get the small bowel up to the new pouch can open over time causing other parts of the bowel to become kinked in the openings and thus blocked. This usually requires further surgery to repair.

Cardiac problems: The greatest risk is in patients who are the most overweight, or who have cardiac disease. Over time the heart of the obese patient enlarges and is at greater risk for problems such as heart attacks. Patients with abnormal EKGs before surgery, or patients at higher risk due to other factors may need further studies to evaluate for cardiac disease prior to surgery.

Ulcers in the pouch: Ulcers can develop in the pouch, or at the connection of the pouch to the small bowel. This can be caused by ingestion of ibuprofen (Motrin®), aspirin, NSAIDs (nonsteroidal anti inflammatories), use of steroids, smoking, or consumption of alcohol. We advise our patients to avoid all of these ulcer-promoting medications. Some believe use of these drugs may increase the risk of erosion in Lap-Band® patients but most Lap-Band® patients can take some ant-inflammatory medications. Usually, with avoidance of ulcerogenic (ulcer-causing) meds, and use of appropriate treatment medications, ulcers can be cured. Rarely, surgery is needed for nonresponsive ulcers at the connection of the stomach and small bowel (marginal ulcers).

Cancer: There is no significant evidence that RYGB or Lap-Band® increase the risk of cancer in the stomach. In fact, stomach cancer risk may be lessened as a result of decreased acid production, and less contact between the stomach and cancer-causing edible agents like nitrosamines, which are ingested in burned meats. (Notice to my Father-in-law who likes "burned to a crisp" steak.) The "mini" RYGB procedure may increase the risk of esophageal-stomach cancer if the acid or bile reflux is significant and not well controlled. In general, any long-term weight loss actually decreases the risk of some cancers (breast, colon, uterine, prostate for example).

Erosion: The Lap-Band® can erode through the wall of the stomach to the inside of the stomach. This can be difficult to diagnose, as symptoms are vague. An infection at the skin port site may be a clue that infection has spread to the band, because if the band is now in the stomach, it may have become infected as the stomach is not entirely sterile. Sometimes patients will notice some mild abdominal pain, which may also be a subtle clue to band erosion. Band erosion is usually treated by removal of the band, and repair of the stomach were the erosion occurred. Fortunately, this now occurs infrequently.

Slippage: The band of the Lap-Band® can also "slip" so that stomach normally below the band slides up through the band. This can cause swelling and blockage of the band, and patients can develop nausea and vomiting. Difficulty with swallowing or heartburn can also develop. Some patients just don't feel as full as usual. This usually requires surgery to repair, and also occurs less frequently now as the stomach is generally sutured to itself over the top of the band.

Nausea and Vomiting: Nausea and vomiting can occur after any surgery simply in response to the anesthetics. Although rare, swelling at the surgical site from irritation or localized bleeding with a clot can also temporarily block emptying of the pouch or band. Dehydration will also exacerbate nausea and electrolyte changes, which then increase the risk of nausea and vomiting. A negative cycle may thus develop and will require IV fluids and electrolyte replacement. A stricture (tightening of the connection between the stomach and small bowel) can also cause nausea and vomiting and usually presents 3-4 weeks out from surgery. The small bowel and pouch can also develop what is called an "ileus," a condition in which the bowel does not contract normally but "goes to sleep", and therefore empties poorly. This usually improves with time, but occasionally requires temporary medications for treatment.

(See note 22 — citations for statistics on complications from bariatric surgery techniques)

Although these complications occur infrequently, they do occur and it is important to have surgery at a facility that can deal appropriately with potential issues. This is not meant to be a comprehensive list, and if you are seriously considering weight loss surgery, you need to discuss with your doctor the benefits, as well as the potential complications of having surgery so that you are fully informed and comfortable with your level of knowledge. Discuss both the benefits and risks in a manner that is specific to your personal medical condition and history.

While you're reading this book, you should make notes of what *you* consider to be benefits or risks, and tuck them in the back of the book. You should also make notes of questions to ask your surgeon, and lodge them in the book as well. In fact, just take your notes, questions, and the whole book with you every time you go to your doctor's office!

Bariatric surgery offers the best-proven method of long-term weight loss for morbidly obese people. This having been said, one must note that all surgery does have risk, including the risk of death. Bariatric surgery is no different, although it does favorably compare to many "common" surgeries. For instance, the mortality rate associated with knee and hip replacement surgery is higher than for typical bariatric cases.[23]

The risk/benefit ratio for bariatric surgery is better than most surgery offered today. How many surgeries can decrease the risk of cancer, improve diabetes, high blood pressure, sleep apnea, arthritis, stress urinary incontinence, acid reflux, and decrease the overall risk of death? In addition, how many surgeries can dramatically improve quality of life while improving medical problems?

A recent landmark study revealed that bariatric surgery lead to an 89% reduction in the relative risk of death as opposed to those morbidly obese patients who had no surgery![24] Another meta-analysis (evaluation of multiple studies), showed that bariatric surgery not only decreases mortality rate, but also decreases the risk of developing new health-related conditions and reduces healthcare utilization and direct health care costs.[25]

In fact, the following co-morbid conditions can be significantly improved and sometimes even eliminated with the utilization of weight loss surgery (excluding Lap-Band®).[26] In fact, no other therapy has produced such durable and complete control of diabetes mellitus.[27]

Hypertension (high blood pressure)	*78.5%*
Type II Diabetes	*86%*
Obstructive Sleep Apnea	*85.7%*
Hyperlipidemia (high cholesterol)	*70%*
Gastroesophageal Reflux Disease	*98%*
Asthma	*Not studied*

TABLE 3.1 — Co-morbidity Improvement Statistics Following Bariatric Surgery

For Lap-Band® patients, studies show the following percentages of co-morbidity improvement or resolution 36 months following surgery:[28]

Hypertension	*48%*
Type II Diabetes	*66%*
Obstructive Sleep Apnea	*33%*
Hyperlipidemia	*65.5%*
Gastroesophageal Reflux	*87%*
Asthma	*81.8%*

TABLE 3.2 — Co-morbidity Improvement Statistics Following Adjustable Gastric Banding (Lap-Band®)

(Results may appear lower because weight loss is generally slower with the Lap-Band® procedure.)

Surgery, however, is not a quick fix. It's not taking the "easy" way out. Patients who have surgery are given a tool — a way to lose weight like they have never before possessed, but they still have to work hard to change their habits and mindset.

As I tell my patients: it's a tool, and it's no different than a hammer or a screwdriver. You can either use the screwdriver to tighten screws, or you can intentionally poke your eye out with it. You can use the hammer to drive nails, or you can whack yourself in the knee. You choose. It's no good to you if you're not using it for the purpose for which it was intended. Patients must use the tool properly to obtain optimal results.

At our center we discuss the "pouch tools," and teach the ways to use the surgical pouch to achieve optimal weight loss. Achieving optimal weight loss means patients should avoid drinking during meals, because the food in the small pouch can be "flushed out" with liquids so the pouch can be filled again. It is important to drink fluid approximately 15-20 minutes before a meal, and then to wait until one hour afterward to drink again.

Liquids with calories must be avoided at all costs as these will slide down through the pouch and give no sense of fullness, yet increase caloric intake. Patients need good behavioral modification support, emotional support, regular exercise, and good nutrition to achieve optimal weight loss after bariatric surgery.

Working with a comprehensive-multidisciplinary team is the best way for a patient to achieve an overall lifestyle change and maintain a healthy weight and life. A patient needs to meet with dietitians, behaviorists, exercise physiologists, and bariatric internists to truly have the best opportunity for maximal weight loss and better health.

Patients should seek surgeons with bariatric experience and proper board certification, who offer comprehensive, multidisciplinary treatment and life-long follow-up. I believe patients are better off finding surgeons who are not "dabbling" in the bariatric area. To be properly familiar with this field of medicine, weight loss surgery should comprise at least 50% of a surgeon's practice. In addition, when evaluating a bariatric surgeon, evidence of regular continuing medical education, and active membership in outstanding bariatric medical societies (ASBS, IFSO) is highly recommended.

A bariatric surgeon's post-operative follow-up should consist of several appointments, not just one. We like to see our patients at two weeks, four weeks, six weeks, three months, six months, and a year after surgery, and at least annually thereafter. It's important for your doctors to periodically monitor your blood levels, nutrition, weight, and other medical issues.

You should not stop being the bariatric surgeon's patient when you come out of the operating room, and of course, you should be having this procedure done in a hospital, not in an outpatient surgical center. (An exception to this rule applies in cases where Lap-Band® procedures are performed by experienced surgeons on lower risk patients.)

Additionally, surgeons and internists should provide good pre-surgical care as well. Medical tests that may need to be run prior to weight loss surgery include: a sleep study, an echocardiogram or heart stress test, and gastrointestinal scope (EGD), an abdominal ultrasound, an ultrasound of the legs, blood tests, diabetes testing, a colon cancer screening if over 50 years old, or a pap smear and mammogram. If you meet with a physician who does not recommend *at least* one of these tests, no matter your age, you should probably look for another physician.

Also, female patients should be aware that pregnancy is not recommended for at least 18 months post surgery. Although that is the recommendation, we have had patients who have become pregnant as early as two weeks after surgery! (I'll give you a moment to digest that little factoid.) It should be noted that this is in direct contradiction of medical advice.

Pregnancy can be managed while the major portion of the weight loss is occurring (the first six months post-operatively), but the patient's nutrition, blood levels, and other medical issues must be very closely monitored. Often a high risk OB specialist is recommended.

And speaking of pre-natal care, it is of the utmost importance that *all* patients having weight loss surgery with a malabsorption component understand that you will have to take vitamins every day for the *rest of your life*. We highly recommend a pre-natal vitamin. Yes, MEN too!! (Men will always get a few odd looks at the pharmacy when they pick up their pre-natal vitamins – especially month after month!)

Why a "pre-natal" vitamin? Because it contains higher concentrations of the nutrients needed to sustain the body than regular vitamins, and it's easier than taking a whole bunch of vitamins at once to get the same effect. Weight Loss surgery patients need the extra calcium, vitamin D, iron, potassium, folic acid, and vitamin B12. All of these are critical in the development of a fetus, and are also critical to the good nutrition of weight loss surgery patients. Overall, these vitamins will help prevent vitamin and mineral deficiencies that can develop after surgery.

The stomach and its acids are essential in helping to absorb vitamin B12 in particular, a nutrient critical for formation of new hemoglobin, the building block for red blood cells. An RYGB changes the stomach's environment such that it is more difficult for the body to absorb vitamin B12 in food. Taking a vitamin containing B12 is essential to allow the body to avoid anemia (low hemoglobin).

Additionally, iron and calcium are primarily absorbed in the first part of the small bowel, which is the part that is bypassed after RYGB surgery. Patients who experience chronic blood loss during menstruation, or from bleeding hemorrhoids should stay in close contact with their doctor as they may require extra iron. Additional calcium will likely be necessary, and can be taken orally in vitamin supplement form.

Not only are they formulated with higher concentrations of essential nutrients, pre-natal vitamins are also highly absorbable because of chelation (kee-lation). Many common over the counter vitamins have extremely poor absorbability. Maximum absorbability is necessary as the pouch does not usually have much acid to assist in breaking down the tablets and making the vitamins more absorbable.

The bariatric procedures that are primarily malabsorptive in nature, cause significantly more electrolyte and vitamin deficiencies than do the procedures being used more often today. Fortunately, most of these procedures are not performed any more. The possibility of vitamin and nutritional deficiencies, and the related effects on the body's systems emphasizes the importance of having life long follow up after bariatric surgery.

Assuming vitamin and nutritional deficiencies are prevented, on average, RYGB patients will lose approximately 70% of their extra weight in the first year to year and a half after surgery. Lap-Band® procedure patients will lose approximately 50-60% of the total weight they have to lose over 2-3 years.[29]

After about six weeks to approximately six months, which we call the "honeymoon period" (because you can literally sleep the time away without significant hunger and the weight will come off), weight loss slows down, and you must be ready to really kick in those revised habits and lifestyle changes or the weight can eventually come back.

There are three main reasons why patients stop losing or regain weight after RYGB surgery. The first is that the pouch can stretch. The older pouches were larger and incorporated a part of the stomach called the "fundus" which we now know stretches, causing the pouch to hold more food. Sometimes the older stretched pouches were surgically revised to remove the stretched fundus portion. As a result of the number of revisions, pouches are now made smaller, and are made to avoid the fundus as much as possible.

A second reason for weight gain can be related to stretching of the opening from the pouch. The ideal opening of the connection is between 12 and 15mm. As the opening widens, food passes through faster and easier, and does not cause as much of a feeling of fullness. Some surgeons place bands around the opening at the time of the original surgery to prevent this stretching, but these bands can erode or cause excessive tightening of the connection. A procedure called *sclerotherapy* which involves injecting an irritant through an endoscope around the widened opening resulting in tightening of the opening is showing some promise in dealing with this problem.

The last main reason for weight gain is maladaptive eating. If one does not use the proper "pouch tools" such as avoiding fluids during meals or avoidance of liquids with calories, weight gain will usually result. The surgery "tool" must be used properly to achieve the best weight loss and develop a long-term healthy lifestyle.

Commitment to lifetime change is critical to maintaining the weight loss. You'll still have to work just as hard mentally and physically to get the weight off and keep it off, as you did without surgery, but with surgery you will have a far greater chance of keeping it off. The body will lose most of the weight in the beginning, but it's up to you to get it the rest of the way, and keep it healthy.

Incidentally, the body will know when to stop losing weight. It may stop for a short time several times along the way (to sort of re-set itself), but it will eventually come to a basic stop. It is the rare person who actually doesn't stop losing weight, and in those unusual cases we reverse our pouch tool techniques to encourage more caloric intake.

We would encourage the use of liquid protein drinks that slide through the pouch, for example. The more malabsorptive procedures (the Distal RYGB, the biliopancreatic diversion, and the duodenal switch) do have a higher incidence of malnutrition, and sometimes additional surgery is required to allow for more intestinal surface to absorb calories, especially protein.[30]

Although at first it will seem like the weight is really dropping off, it will slow down, and for that patients must be prepared. It is important to note that this is a *process*. It is a process that occurs over a fairly long time period, so don't try to rush it. Trust me, and trust Julie and Karen when we tell you that it will fly by all on its own. Let your body move on its own time schedule, and that includes plateaus, slow downs, and "shrinks" (a term they'll define for you later in the book.). It took you many years to put on this weight, so it's going to take at least a year, and maybe two or three years to completely get it off.

And on that note, don't rush to plastic surgery. I recommend that my patients wait at least 18 months before having plastic surgery to have skin removed. The body needs time to shrink and adjust to its new size and shape. Plastic surgery for skin removal is *not* necessary in all patient cases. It should be evaluated on a case-by-case basis. We'll discuss this more in Chapter Fourteen.

So, in the long run, how effective is bariatric surgery, really? Well, to quote a lawyer friend of mine (Julie!), "*it depends.*" It depends on how old you are, how much you weighed before surgery, the type of procedure you had done, how motivated you were to stick to your lifestyle changes, what you eat, how much you exercise, the level of emotional support you have, your overall health, and whether or not you take your pre-natal vitamins. How's that for a non-commital answer?!

Success in bariatric surgery is commonly defined as achieving loss of 50% or more of excess body weight, and maintaining that level for at least five years.[31] I would add that success could also be rated by the overall improvement in the patient's health and weight related medical conditions. Remember, for (non-surgical) medical weight loss programs, success is usually defined as loss of 10-15% of extra weight.[32] As surgeons we prefer to have at least one half or more of the extra weight dissipate and remain gone.

Patients with higher initial Body Mass Indexes (BMIs) tend to lose more total weight. Patients with lower initial BMIs tend to lose a greater percentage of their excess weight, and may be more likely to come closer to their ideal body weight.[33] Patients with type II diabetes tend to show less overall excess weight loss than patients without type II diabetes.[34] One study shows patients can maintain a 50-60% loss of excess weight 10 to 14 years after bariatric surgery and approximately 50% off for 20 years.[35] Patients also have significant improvement in their quality of life. Basic things like fitting into seats, walking, and general hygiene become immeasurably easier with weight loss.

If anyone can come up with a non-surgical, medical weight loss program with significantly better long-term results than the measly 0-2% of dieters who keep their weight off long-term, they should be eligible for a Pulitzer Prize in medicine! Until then we need to be painfully honest about the adverse sequelae of obesity, and the poor results of our present dietary and medical interventions.

The risks of weight loss surgery should not be downplayed, but neither should the risks of morbid obesity. It is not intellectually honest to downplay the significant problems related to obesity and the lack of success with medical approaches to weight loss, while playing-up the risks of bariatric surgery. The reality now is that surgery offers the best-documented long-term way for morbidly obese patients to lose weight and become healthier. But if you prefer to ignore the facts, I have some great lemon extract on sale for only $169.99. If you act today, I might even throw in a Gin-soo knife that can cut through pennies.

Even cowards can endure hardship;
only the brave can endure suspense.

MIGNON MCLAUGHLIN

Chapter Four

SCRAMPS, AND STRICTURE, AND HICCUPS, OH MY!!

Julie M. Janeway
Karen J. Sparks

Okay. You've just read all the medical information about weight loss surgery, and you may still be finding yourself a bit curious about some of the potential complications and after-effects that can result. Well, we've decided to write a little about our experiences with complications and after-effects to help ease that curiosity.

But before we get into that, just a quick word on the topic of dealing with post-surgical complications. First, you may not have any complications, but you will have after-effects, so be prepared. You'll understand the difference between them as you read through the chapter.

Second, don't be afraid of complications because the doctors aren't afraid of them. Trust that you've chosen a physician who is more than competent and capable of handling anything that comes up, and that he or she is prepared and ready to appropriately deal with whatever you may experience.

Third, what other people had, you might not have; but… you might. Each person is very different, and there's no predicting what can happen. Not even your surgeon can predict what will occur or not occur. Just wait and see. We hope (knock on wood) you won't have any complications to speak of, and your after-effects will be mild, and more humorous than annoying or painful.

Fourth, be prepared to deal with whatever comes your way. It's part of the package. Remember that you've already dealt with so many more issues, so much more pain, and far worse things than whatever complications you may experience as a result of this surgery. Just grit your teeth and persevere. Chances are excellent that all will work out well in the end.

Finally, don't lose perspective, or your sense of humor. Keeping everything in perspective and relative to the entire timeline of the process is key. Your sense of humor is so important in getting you through tough times. If you start to lose your sense of humor, make sure you turn to your support network for help in fighting through the rough patches one day, or one hour, or even one minute at a time.

Now, back to complications and after-effects. We've chosen to organize this chapter by using little subheadings to keep it simple and easy to find things for later reference. We've also indicated under each subheading who had the issue, and therefore who's writing about it. If both of us had it, then it's generally me (Julie) who's writing about it. That probably means Karen's off teaching a class somewhere. But, if she alone had the issue, then she's recording her experiences for posterity all by herself.

The following are the experiences we had with our surgeries, and you may have different experiences, or not experience these things at all. The best we can tell you is prepare for the worst, and hope for the best.

POTENTIAL COMPLICATIONS

STRICTURE
Julie

Well, we might as well start with the most common complication of weight loss surgery. Dr. Baker has explained stricture to you in the previous chapter. If you've already forgotten, go back and look it up. I'll wait……..dum dee dum dum, da dee dum dee dee……… Got it? Good.

I had a stricture, which is statistically the most common complication after RYGB surgery. The stricture first occurred within a week or so following gastric bypass. I couldn't get the protein drinks down, and it eventually got to the point that I couldn't get water or any other liquid down either. The less protein and fluid I took in, the more dehydrated and starved my body got, the more tired and sick I was, and the less I cared about even trying to get anything in.

I was fairly stubborn about all this, and didn't want to bother Dr. Baker. After all, he is a very busy man, and I thought he'd think I was just a whiny, wimpy patient. So, I just sucked it up and hoped it would pass.

When I went back for my two week follow-up appointment, I broke down and told him what was going on. Of course, he couldn't believe I'd waited so long to tell anybody, but never once did he scold or berate me. He simply dove right into taking care of it, and assured me it would be okay. After examining me, listening to me cry, and asking me a number of questions, he informed me that he suspected I had a stricture and he immediately scheduled an endoscopy.

An endoscopy is a procedure that involves sending a long tube with a camera in the tip down your throat and into your stomach. The doctors can have a lovely little look around, and in the event things have constricted because of swelling or spasm, they can send a little balloon type device down there and pop it open again. All in all, it's not unlike snaking a drain. They reel it down, have a look around, push through the blockage, and reel it back up. Voila! You can dump stuff down the drain and it will run right out to the sewer system again.

So, Dr. Kemmeter from MMPC® took me in for an endoscopy. Now, for those of you who've never had an endoscopy, I will tell you that the worst part of having one is really getting the I.V. in. I was none too happy with the concept of having a complication at all, let alone having a stricture because it involved having another procedure done under sedation, which meant another I.V.

Because of my car accident, and by my personal calculations, in the previous three years I'd had about three million, four hundred sixty two thousand, seven hundred and fourteen needle and I.V. sticks, give or take a hundred or so. Also, for such a big person, I had virtually non-existent veins, and add to that the fact that I was massively dehydrated, and you can get the picture on what a pure joy it was to try and have an I.V. started.

After a few-more-than-several attempts to get the I.V. started, I not-so-calmly reminded them that I was a "hard stick," and suggested that they might find someone who was trained to start pediatric I.V.s (a little trick I learned when in the hospital with my car accident). The theory is: if you can start one on a preemie, chances are you can get one on me. I'd been a good sport to that point, but you can only play pincushion for so long. To their credit, the nurses quickly found someone who had just that sort of training, and she came down and slapped that puppy right in on the first try. I promised her a large bequest of jewelry in my will.

Following the I.V. incident, the rest was a breeze. They give you some sedation meds to start calming you down (or maybe it's just me…I don't know), and then they wheel you into the procedure room. It's not really an operating room, it's just sort of like a hospital room with more sterile medical monitors and junk in it. Anyway, they got me situated laying on my side, told me again quickly what they were going to do, then they ran some drugs in the IV, and that was it. I don't remember a thing until they were waking me up in recovery.

In recovery you're pretty groggy. You don't really know where you are or why. They seem to think that getting you to drink something is important, so I complied. Personally, in recovery, I just want to be left alone. Unfortunately they don't think that's an option. They let you lay there for around an hour or so, during which time the doctor comes and talks to you about what he or she found.

At least that's what I'm told. I don't ever remember talking to the doctor because the drugs kind of wipe out your memory for a while after the procedure. (I'm quite sure they were developed by the CIA or something.) But I know I talked to the doctor because my husband, Matt swears I did (unless the CIA got to him too), and I came home with a lovely parting gift of full color before and after pictures of my insides. (I thought lovely parting gifts always included Rice-a-Roni® and Chico-San Rice Cakes®…?)

Interestingly, the color pictures are pretty drastic. It turns out that the opening from my pouch to my roux limb was mostly closed off. Overall, very little was getting through. Hey, it happens. At least they knew how to fix it. And the color photos double as pretty nifty post-modern art pieces if you frame them just right.

So that was my first experience with stricture. Unfortunately it was not my last. My little innards are pretty stubborn, and by a couple of weeks later, the opening had spasmed and strictured closed again. Back to the endoscopy suite I went.

This time I got the pediatric I.V. nurse right off the bat, so I circumvented that drama. Again, Dr. Kemmeter cranked open the stricture. Again I went to recovery. Again, I purportedly talked to the doctor. And again, I came home with another piece for my post-modern art collection.

We were all pretty sure at this point that the opening would stay open, as most people only have to go through this once. I, of course, had to be one of the minority that has to go through it more than once. Apparently my innards are slow learners, and about a month later, I was right back in there having it done again.

Now before I go any further, I feel it necessary to stress that this is highly unusual, but not unheard of. I've already stated that I'm a person who likes to test limitations and boundaries, and apparently so does my gastrointestinal tract. I guess it just wanted to see if it could really get Dr. Kemmeter back in there a third time.

By this point, I had the process down to a science. The I.V. went right in, the procedure went without a hitch, and I got another piece of art for the collection. But before I went under, I did ask Dr. Kemmeter if there was a record for the number of times someone had to undergo this procedure. He declined to tell me in case subconsciously I'd try to break it. I also asked if there was some other measure that could be taken to hold the opening in place, and he assured me that this procedure would do the trick. Turns out he was right. I was third time lucky.

Stricture isn't fun, but it can be dealt with effectively. Many people say they have a mild sore throat for a day or so following the procedure, but I never did. Kudos to Dr. Kemmeter. All I ever had was the need to sleep for 24 hours after each procedure. You are advised to go back to soft and liquid foods for a day or two, but past that you're up and moving around with no issues.

It's a fairly common complication of weight loss surgeries, so don't be shocked if you find yourself in an endoscopy suite afterward. I survived my strictures, and if you find yourself being visited by the stricture fairy, you will too.

BLEEDERS AND BLOOD TRANSFUSIONS
Karen

Although I didn't have all the drama that usually accompanies anything Julie does, I, too, had a surgical complication. My complication involved a blood vessel or something that decided to leak causing a great purplish-red-black bruise on the right side of my torso. Later, we affectionately dubbed it "Lake Michigan" because that was how it was shaped.

My bruise started to form right after surgery, and as I was still enjoying the Morphine ride, I didn't notice, nor did I care. At one point, however, I tried to resituate myself in the bed, and noticed the growing discoloration. I made a mental note, and went back to dream land.

In any hospital, trips to dreamland are only a few minutes long. It's sort of like trying to sleep on the subway, you keep waking up at every stop. In the hospital there's always a nurse or someone else there to check on something or another, or to wake you up to tell you to go to sleep. I know that's a good thing, but let's be honest; it's still annoying.

Anyway, they came in to draw blood, and when the results came back, they noticed my blood counts were low. They took my blood pressure again, and noticed that it had dropped. At that point, I was coherent just long enough to relate to the nurse my notice of "Lake Michigan" before the Morphine had me off on another adventure. (Man I love those little PCA "jeopardy" button things they give you for self-administering pain meds....)

The next thing I remember was Dr. Baker appearing in my room and telling me that he was ordering some blood because my blood level was too low. He mentioned something about a suspected bleeder, and if the transfusion didn't work they'd have to go back in and find it. I mumbled through my Morphine haze that I trusted him completely, and to do whatever he thought he needed to do.

Three units of blood were hung, and my blood pressure slowly started to rise (although I don't know how, as I swear they took at least two units back out in blood samples). I was finally strong enough to have them remove the Foley catheter, and to get up to go to the bathroom.

When I went to the bathroom, I was horrified to see the toilet filled with blood, and quickly assumed I must be bleeding to death. I almost hung myself flailing about grasping for that little rope that calls for the nurse. When he came he told me everything was okay, and that it was actually a good thing because it meant that my body was expelling some of the oozing blood and my bowels were working again. My choices at that point were to believe him, or believe I would be dead in ten minutes. I chose to believe him. Good choice.

The next problem was that my iron had dropped terribly in the process of losing and replacing my blood volume. I had to take liquid iron supplements for weeks after, which is like some sort of court-ordered punishment. I don't care what flavor they try and give it, it still tastes like you're sucking on a metal hanger. I suffered, and I mean SUFFERED through every one of those doses, but eventually that too came to an end.

Finally, my blood levels evened out, and Lake Michigan receded. Today I am just fine, and I've suffered no ill effects from my complications. I owe it all to the fact that I chose a physician who was knowledgeable, on-top of things, and was a person whom I trusted, literally with my life.

Trust is such an important thing in this situation. It wasn't the most pleasant thing I've ever gone through, but neither was it the worst. It wasn't optimal, but it was do-able. I got through it one minute at a time, and I never looked back.

THRUSH
Julie

Hi. It's me, back again. Yes, I had this one too. For those of you who don't know what Thrush is, its real medical name is *Candidiasis*, and it is a really nifty little infection that you generally get in your mouth. The way they diagnose it is by having you open your mouth really wide. They look at your tongue, and if it's coated with this icky white stuff that kind of looks like a thin schmeer of cream cheese, they know you have it. Babies get Thrush a lot. It's not exactly lethal, but it can be life-threatening if it gets into your system and works its way to your heart or other major organs.

As I told you earlier, I was pretty sick just from dealing with the effects of my stricture, and my immune system was fairly defenseless at this point because I hadn't eaten anything in weeks. I was trying to drink skim milk because at least it had some nutrients, and it contains a high amount of protein per ounce. Never mind that I'm lactose intolerant; it was "damn the torpedoes, full steam ahead" in trying to find some form of protein that I could get in, and keep in.

The use of any antibiotics (like you get before and after surgery) can predispose toward developing Thrush. Once your normal system flora (normal good bacteria) is affected, the microbe check and balance system gets out of whack. This then allows the infection to grow unchecked The problem was that I didn't know I had it, and because I was so weak and tired, it just flew down my esophagus and invaded my gastrointestinal system.

I found it ironic that nothing else could get through the stricture, but that nasty little infection just drove right through like a Mack truck. The internal Thrush infection just made matters a little worse, but as soon as I went for another check-up with Dr. Baker, he found it, wrote a prescription, again listened to me cry, and again assured me I was going to be okay.

The treatment for Thrush is generally a course of Nystatin®, Diflucan®, Clotrimazole®, or Fluconazole®. Ladies, if these look familiar to you, it's because you're right, they are the same drugs administered for yeast infections at the other end of the body.

Thrush is a form of yeast infection, and it is generally treated either topically or internally (orally) for a period of about ten days or so. In my case, I was prescribed liquid Nystatin® in a pretty hefty dosage, with instructions to hold it in my mouth for about thirty seconds, swish it around, and then swallow it. I had to do this four times a day; which meant four times a day I made myself wildly sick trying to get unsick.

My Thrush was particularly persistent, but as it began to beat a retreat, I got better and moved to a second course of treatment that was Diflucan® in pill form, once a day. When the stricture issue eased up and I could get some normal food in, the Thrush was finally terminated. Moral of the story: You can flush the Thrush!! It's not so hot to have, but in the greater scheme of things, pretty low on the "Why Me, God?" list.

Neither one of us had any of the other five major types of complications. They are infection, pneumonia or lung collapse, pulmonary embolism, hernia, and bowel leakage or obstruction. Dr. Baker has talked about each of these potential complications in the previous chapter, so we believe it would be redundant to address them again; plus, we don't have any good stories to tell about them.

Suffice it to say, if you get one of these complications, you simply have to treat it like any other, and face it head on knowing you are under the care of a capable, competent, and kind surgeon who won't let you fall through the cracks. To quote a phrase, "Just pull up your big girl panties and deal with it!" (Apologies to the men reading this…)

Now on to the more fun part of this chapter: AFTER-EFFECTS!! Yeah! Everyone who has some form of weight loss surgery is going to have one or more of these weird after-effects. This is the stuff nobody tells ya, folks!!! You never hear people talk about this stuff on talk shows or the Discovery Channel®!! This is the everyday weirdness you'll deal with if you have weight loss surgery — plain and simple. It's not horrible, it's just weird. It's not deadly, it's just weird. Sometimes it's painful, but mostly……. it's just weird. It's not an all-inclusive list, just a sampling of some of the weird stuff that can happen. We've organized this section of the chapter the same way we organized the complications section, except we're going to write about them in the order in which they appeared. So without any further adieu, here they are.

POTENTIAL AFTER-EFFECTS

BLOATING AND TORSO PAIN
Julie and Karen

Ouch!! We both remember this one quite vividly. Most people experience this, and if you don't, well then they've got you on WAY too much Morphine! If you have weight loss surgery done laparoscopically the surgeon needs to fill your chest and abdominal cavity up with air so he or she can have room to maneuver things like the instruments and your liver. You know how you can spill a small glass of water, and as soon as it's out of the cup it's like a flood of biblical proportions? Well that's sort of the same principle behind how much air they put in you to do these surgeries.

The small incisions that are made in order to do the surgery are pretty well plugged up with the instruments, so not much air really escapes. When they're done the re-plumbing of your gastrointestinal tract, they take the instruments out and close the little holes. What results is basically what we like to call "the beach ball effect."

Remember as a kid (or more recently as a parent) blowing up those cheap plastic beach balls? You huff and puff, and huff and puff, and suck wind, and huff and puff, and wonder if the stupid thing will ever fill up all they way… and then you move to plug it and some of the air escapes. By this time, however, you're so tired of huffing and puffing that you don't much care as long as the darn thing floats (and if you're a parent, that the kids play with it and get lost).

The ball gets some play and is tossed around a bit, but mostly the kids just let it float around the pool. Eventually, the air just leaks out on its own, the ball goes flat, and then it goes wherever one sock always goes in the dryer. (Where is that?)

Anyway, this is pretty much what happens with the air they stuff inside you, except for the huffing and puffing part… I hope. They toss you around a bit in surgery, but then you just kind of float around while you're recovering, and eventually the air just leaks out, and you go flat. If you end up going where the one sock always goes, could you call us and let us know where that is? Thanks.

But we digress…. The point of telling you all this is that while the proverbial ball is going flat, it tends to be a little painful. You will most likely feel as though somebody broke a couple of ribs in surgery, and you'll most likely ask someone to check and see if they did. They didn't. Trust us. You'll probably feel like your rib cage is burning a little, but that's more than likely just some inflammation of the muscle tissue and the fascia. Also, it will feel as though if you roll over, all your guts will fall out. You can roll over, gently, as soon as your doctor says it's all right to do so. They won't fall out. Trust us.

So that's the bad news, but the good news is two-fold: 1) you don't have to deal with this for long; and, 2) your doctor can give you medication to help you deal with it. These sensations only last for about a week to ten days on the whole, with each day getting a little better. Well…except the second and third days; they're pretty bad. It's kind of like working out; you're not really sore until the second day after the workout. Get it? If you have a good doctor (and you will), he or she will make sure that you have appropriate medications to help you deal with this discomfort. Julie and Karen's Prognosis: Icky, but totally survivable.

PAPER CUTS
Julie and Karen

If you've had a laparoscopic procedure, then you're going to end up with six little incisions about a half-inch long each. They'll most likely just put steristrips (little

—TOO MUCH AIR—

bandaid like things) over them to keep them closed, or they might plunk in one or two stitches under the steristrips. Either way, you're probably going to have six little wounds. How much do they hurt? Well, we call them paper cuts, and that's about as much as they hurt.

You know when you get a nasty paper cut, like from a file folder or cardboard? That's about what they feel like. After about five days, you really don't feel them anymore, assuming they don't get infected or something. But from our experience, and from the experiences of others we've talked to, you'll probably have one that will just wake up and poke you every once in a while, just to let you know it's there.

It will probably be one of the paper cuts toward the side of your torso, or the uppermost one in the front, as they seem to be the ones that rub most against clothes. For guys, the list could also include the one in your belly button if the waistband of your pants sits right there. Julie and Karen's Prognosis: Pretty low on the annoyance list. You'll recover.

ALLERGIES
Julie and Karen

There's a strange phenomenon that occurs in hospitals: the creation of allergies where none existed before. Both Karen and I developed, or maybe just discovered that we are allergic to certain types of pain medication while in hospitals. I am allergic to Dilaudid® and Demerol®, and Karen found out she is allergic to Morphine (despite the fun rides it takes her on).

It's not like you generally discover a life-threatening type allergy, although you could. You will generally discover the kind of allergy that just sort of drives you nuts by making you itch so bad you could take a steel barbeque grill brush to your hide! Karen's is technically an allergy because she itches something awful, but she doesn't break out in hives. I break out in hives and welts, so I know it's an allergy. I know that if I get hives and I don't attend to the situation promptly, my eyes and throat will begin to swell closed, and then it's not a good place to be.

Allergies are generally nothing major, just tell somebody you're uncomfortable or itchy and they'll give you some antihistamines and change your pain meds. Note: if you begin to break out in hives, if anything begins to swell up, or you can't breath, call for help immediately. Julie and Karen's Prognosis: Generally, no big deal. Annoying but endurable.

REVERSE HICCUPS
Julie and Karen

Now this little critter is an animal of a different sort. It's kind of unique to bariatric surgery patients, or maybe even just gastric bypass patients. All we know is that it's a very bizarre experience and condition, and it doesn't seem to go away.

As the name we've given it suggests, it feels like a form of hiccup (or hiccough for our European readers). When you have a normal hiccup, you kind of draw in air ridiculously fast. It's like there's a quick spasm, and then you're sucking in air.

But with a reverse hiccup, you still have the hiccup part, but from the point of the spasm in your gut, food and/or air also moves the opposite way through your intestines. That's the part that hurts. So it's like you're hiccupping in two directions at once. It sounds like this: HIC! OW!!

Dr. Baker tells me this is part of peristalsis which happens every time you eat. Peristalsis is the process of pushing food through the intestinal tract. Apparently the small bowel is always contracting, almost like a pump, but now it's hooked up high to the new pouch. The closeness of the small bowel to the upper abdomen causes more noticeable "growling" bowel sounds, and hiccups (involuntary contraction of the diaphragm) may affect the peristalsis of the pouch and small bowel such that the strange "OW" sensation occurs. Dr. Baker also noted that much more study, however, is needed to evaluate this theory.

If you have reverse hiccups too often, there's medication that can be prescribed to stop some of the spasms Other than that, it's one of those weird things that you'll just deal with after surgery. We have no explanation for why this occurs only after surgery, but it does. And that's all we have to say about that. Julie and Karen's Prognosis: Weird, but you'll live.

AIR BUBBLES
Julie and Karen

Let us tell you right now, from the moment you come out of surgery your biggest enemy on the planet is air. To clarify: air is bad, unless you're breathing it. Air bubbles can feel like you've swallowed a VW Bug. They will cause unbelievable intestinal cramps that will have you twisting and contorting like a Cirque du Soleil performer. Air is to be avoided at all costs.

Avoiding gastrointestinal air intake involves eating slowly, chewing food very well, and avoiding all foods that cause air to enter the system. Also, not laughing while drinking something, because you tend to suck in a lot of air through your nose and then you swallow it. If you do this, you'll be experiencing the after-effect we discuss in the next chapter. (Voices of experience talking here....)

Most people swallow air while eating, especially if you are gulping. The air is generally stored in the stomach, which is usually a reservoir of sufficient size for it. After surgery, the reservoir is no longer attached to the esophagus, and only a small pouch exists to hold both air and food, thus the bloating and painful effect of gas is exponentially increased. To prevent this, you should avoid foods like broccoli, cucumbers, onions, soda pop, carbonated water, milk, peppers, bread, rice, and sometimes beans. There are others, but you'll have to make your own list of no-no's as you experience them. Air is pain. Air is your enemy.

If you are engaged by the enemy, your only survival tactic is to attempt to work it out, or wait it out. Some people say Beano® helps with the air issue, but that hasn't been our experience. If you want to try it, consult with your doctor first. Medications containing Simethicone® such as Gas-X® may be helpful. Once you experience the kind of air bubble pain we're talking about, you'll learn to avoid the foods that cause the explosion or implosion of your intestines. Julie and Karen's Prognosis: Avoidable, manageable, but tolerable if necessary.

REPEATED BURPING
Karen

Related to the air bubble issue, is the issue of what we have termed Repeated Rhythmic Burping (RRB). Again, this is associated with peristalsis, but what results are repeated burps that occur in an evenly spaced rhythmic pattern. They may go on for hours. It sounds like this: Burp. Burp. Burp. Burp. Burp. (multiply this times eighty-four more lines of text). It *doesn't* sound like this: Burp. Buuuurrrrrpppp!! Aaaahhhh!!

Neither one of us can figure out where all the air comes from. Julie and I can eat the same meal, eat the same amount over the same amount of time, and I'll end up with RRB, while she only gets two (and almost always two) reverse hiccups. What results is that if we're shopping when this occurs, I'm stuck in the car trying to deal with the RRB, and she's already scoped through the clearance and sale racks, and she gets all the good bargains. Meanwhile, I'm digging through my purse looking for the prescription the doctor gave me to deal with the RRB. Not fair!!

This type of thing can be headed off with a script for Misoprostol®, or it's generic version Cytotec®. This medication helps to protect the lining of the stomach, but also helps to improve emptying of the pouch, which assists in moving along some of the gas. The prescription can be taken two ways. You can take it before eating, or after the burping starts. I can't really identify what's going to set it off, and I don't want to take the pills if I'm not having an issue, so I wait and take it after the RRB strikes.

I've eliminated the foods we listed previously in the "Air Bubbles" section, and many more. Sometimes I can eat a particular food and I have no problems. Other times I can eat the exact same food, and I get RRB. Go figure! But, generally about ten minutes after I take the medication, the RRB subsides. Unfortunately, that's right about the time Julie gets back in the car with the great sale shoes, and the other stuff that would have rightfully been mine were it not for the RRB ambush!! Julie and Karen's Prognosis: Annoying, strange, and totally unfair in a shopping environment.

SNEEZING WHEN YOU EAT
Julie and Karen

This has happened to both of us, but it happens to Karen far more regularly, and with far more ferocity. This one has no medical explanation we can find. It's a once-in-a-while phenomenon and is more weird than anything.

Occasionally, you'll eat something too quickly, and the bite will have been too big. It will kind of get stuck on the way down, but it's not like you're choking or anything. While you are swallowing and trying to get it to go down, you may find that your body just creates an immediate sneeze right out of thin air.

It won't be just any old sneeze; it'll be a massive, tropical storm type sneeze, and the next thing you know the food is unstuck and moving on. Don't know what to tell you about this one folks, but we've both experienced it, as have others we've talked to, and we're just chalking this one up to the weird column. Julie and Karen's Prognosis: Whatever…

FOOD INTOLERANCES
Julie and Karen

Again, we're sure there's some long, involved medical explanation for this that includes a dissertation on enzymes, amino acids, and peptides, but all we know is that it happens to everybody who has weight loss surgery.

Every person we've ever talked to has had some sort of food intolerance issue. For some people it's immediate lactose intolerance, for others it's eggs, red meat, chicken, fish, or things that contain caffeine. It can be anything, even something you've eaten a million times -- even something that's good for you like fruit, or a particular vegetable like corn or cauliflower.

We have no way of telling you what foods you'll be able to tolerate, and what ones you won't, and neither can your doctor, dietitian, or the Psychic Friends Network. This one you do on your own.

Our rule is if it makes you sick twice on two different days, separated by at least three weeks, then give it up for a while. The doctors and dietitians will tell you to wait a couple of months and try again. Some foods you'll choose to try again, like apples, or bananas, or bread. Others will have made you so sick, you turn a strange teal color just thinking about them (see our stories in the Auto Eject Chapter), and for those foods… well, maybe not so much….

We thought it important to warn you that this was coming, because it could be something as unnoticeable as black pepper, or garlic, or oregano. You'll have to experiment. Everything is an experiment!!! We should all get honorary food science degrees for dealing with this stuff!! Consider yourself warned. Now you're on your own. Julie and Karen's Prognosis: Irritating, but you'll live to tell the tale.

GALLBLADDER ISSUES
Karen

This potential after-effect of weight loss is no fun. Really, really, hope this doesn't happen, but if it does, know that it can be dealt with effectively and efficiently.

About two months after my gastric bypass surgery I began to develop stabbing pain in my side, which quickly progressed into unusual bouts of vomiting and nausea that weren't necessarily related to eating. The first time I felt the debilitating pain, I was bending down and to the right to pick something up in my kitchen, and ARRRGGHHH!, I was virtually blinded with pain, and I couldn't straighten up for about ten minutes. I thought, "That's not good…."

The second time it happened was about a week later, when I was sitting in my office. I dropped my pen, and when I leaned down and to the right to get it, I almost fell off the chair in abject agony. When I could finally straighten up, I wiped away the tears, and called Dr. Baker for help.

He scheduled an appointment for two days hence, and ordered an immediate ultrasound of my gallbladder. When I got to Dr. Baker's office, the results of the ultrasound were in, and it turned out that I had one big 2-centimeter gallstone fouling things up. Dr. Baker said it had to come out. I was profoundly glad. At that point I would have let him take an arm and a leg to get rid of that piercing pain.

Surgery was booked for about a week later. In the meantime, Dr. Baker gave me some medication to deal with the symptoms. It helped with the level of pain, but not only did the symptoms not go away, they continued to get worse.

Although the medication was dealing with the level of pain, pain became a more frequent visitor, and it brought with it its little friends "nausea" and "vomiting." At first I thought I was just eating foods that I wasn't ready for, but it turns out that most of my hurling episodes were gallbladder related. The most memorable event came one very cold night after we'd tried to eat some fajitas at a Mexican restaurant (a stupid endeavor in its own right...).

Without grossing anybody out, I spent over an hour standing in a parking lot, in the freezing cold, separating myself from what food I'd managed to consume. I was so sick I couldn't hold my head up, and it was almost three hours before I could get in the car and drive home. That night, the 45-minute ride home also included two unscheduled pit stops to separate myself from food I don't think I'd even eaten yet.

A week later I was in surgery. Interestingly, they take the gallbladder out laparoscopically when they can, and they use some of the same holes from your gastric bypass surgery. You also get two new ones about the same size. (Hey, what's a few more paper cuts between friends...?)

I was home the next day, and off work about three more only because I wanted the break. I haven't had any trouble since, and it was really no big deal to go in and have it removed. Once you've been in surgery, it takes away all the fear of the unknown. Note, gallbladder issues are the result of the weight loss, not the result of surgery per se. It's a potential after-effect, not a usual or direct complication of surgery.

Don't fear this potential after-effect. It happens to many people, and good surgeons will deal with it in a timely and competent manner. Julie and Karen's Prognosis: What doesn't kill you makes you stronger.

THERMOSTAT ISSUES
Julie and Karen

This one happens to almost everyone who has a drastic weight loss. When you were heavy, you probably dealt with the issue of being hot all the time (or as Karen likes to put it: "bursting into flames.") You were always complaining about being too hot, about people (read here: minions of hell) keeping the heat up too high, and you may never have understood why people whined so much about cold weather because to you it was often a welcome relief.

Remember the agony of hot, humid summer days? Remember standing in the freezer section at the grocery store for an inordinately long time? Remember wondering why skinny people never perspired, or looked like they were roasting like a Jordan almond? Well the reason is that fat is a wonderful insulator. Once you lose the fat, amazingly you're not bursting into flames anymore.

In fact, you should be prepared for just the opposite. Your poor little body is so used to being well insulated that you have to acclimatize all over again. Don't be surprised if now you're the one complaining about how cold you are, or how low people keep their thermostats (heat nazis…), or how unbelievably frigid it is outside. (There have been several occasions we've almost become convinced that a second ice age is here….)

So stock up on sweaters and sweatshirts, and get used to wearing a coat again. In fact, don't be surprised if you own more coats after surgery, than you collectively owned in all your years before surgery.

Note: issues will arise with others in your house or office as a result of your personal thermostat problem. Strangely, others will not find it humorous to discover the thermostat has gone from what appears to be 68 on the dial (ya, right!), to a comfortable and balmy 84. Ladies, your husbands may simply refuse to understand that having a space heater no more than four feet from you at all times is as necessary to life as water and air. Similarly, they're not about to understand or accept that you need more than them to keep you warm at night; at least two additional comforters will be required.

For those of you who live in warmer climates, don't think you'll escape this experience. It will probably just be less drastic. For those of you who live through cold, snowy northern winters, buckle up 'cause it's going to be one arctic-cold ride! Julie and Karen's Prognosis: S-s-s-s-survivable.

SCRAMPS!!
Julie and Karen

"Scramps" is a word that was invented by my nine year-old niece, Meghan. Meghan suffers from a gastrointestinal disorder that has caused her terrible cramps since she was a baby. When she was very little and learning to talk, of course she had a hard time conveying the pain she was in. As she grew and mastered language a little more, she finally learned to tell us when the "scramps" were starting so we could help her head them off, or help her through an episode.

We've adopted Meghan's term "scramps" because the searing, ripping pain that you can get in your legs or torso after a significant amount of weight loss is like "screaming" "cramps," or "scramps." We're not talking about your regular, every day charley horse in your calf here. We're talking about oh-my-good-golly, there must be some horrific netherworld force at work ripping my flesh from my bones, kill me now and spare me this misery – Pain!

We've found virtually no significant medical literature on this phenomenon as it relates to weight loss surgery patients, and we're in the process of convincing several medical researchers to begin a study to help explain exactly what it is, and why and when it occurs.

What goes on here feels like someone is actually ripping the muscles away from the bones in your leg! Additionally, the muscles then spasm, and each segment of your leg from joint to joint may actually twist in a different direction, making it feel as though your leg is being wrung like a dirty mop! Apparently there is a medical term for this: "tetany." We don't care what you call it, it hurts!

Now multiply this by two if you happen to get both legs going at the same time. Somehow, one leg seems to have sympathy for the other, and says, "Hey, if you can't beat 'em, join 'em!" Sometimes the pain and spasm is so bad that you can't even get up to try and walk it out. News flash — this doesn't really work anyway....

Poor Karen gets this quite often. The first time she experienced it, we were away at an academic conference with another professor friend of ours, Judy, who is a nurse. The little college we were teaching for at the time had all of us staying in one hotel room (cheap college...). Karen began experiencing this ungodly pain in her leg. She tried to go out in the hallway and walk it off, but she was limping too badly, and it just got worse.

Judy first suggested putting ice on it, which we tried, but I knew from months of cramps similar to this (after twenty reconstructive surgeries following my car accident), that heat was probably the better way to go. Judy agreed.

I convinced Karen to get into the bathtub, pajamas and all, and I ran quite warm water in the tub as fast as I could. I had Judy massaging Karen's calf in a motion moving only toward the heart, and getting Karen to breath deeply and stop crying.

You have to understand how much this hurts. Karen is a very strong and competent person. You don't get to be an academic Dean of over half a college campus being a whiner or a wimp. If Karen had broken down in tears, I knew we were dealing with cataclysmic pain.

After about an hour and a half, we finally got the pain under control, and got her leg to stop contorting and twisting in multiple directions at the same time. She was cold, wet, and beat up, but over all none-the-worse-for-the-wear. She could still walk, so we called it a success. We'd beaten back the leg scramps! Victory was ours!!

But what is actually worse than the leg pain, is if this occurs in your torso! PAIN! PAIN! PAIN! OW! OW! OW!

About seven months after my surgery I'd lost probably 80 pounds or more, and I was sitting on the couch grading papers. I'd just eaten something for dinner, and about a half hour later I began to feel a little nauseous and uncomfortable, so I lay down on the couch. Immediately after changing positions I began to feel crampy discomfort, but it didn't feel like intestinal cramps. My ribs began to burn from what felt like the underside, and things in my torso just began to hurt.

I stood up and stretched my arms over my head, but that didn't work, and was making it a little worse. So I went and stretched in a doorway by hooking my hands on the upper jamb, and pulling down. That made things exponentially worse, so I lay down on the bed. I was now in a significant amount of pain, but because I'm very good in a crisis, I remained calm and rational about the situation.

Because of my analytical nature, I laid there trying to figure out what could be causing me such pain. I tried to slow my breathing down, but within about ten minutes it became very hard to breathe, and my heart began to race. It felt as though my chest were caving in.

The pain was beginning to overwhelm me. I couldn't lie there anymore, so I got up and tried to walk around the house. I was alone, and since I live out in the country twenty minutes from a hospital, I was starting to get a little worried. I wasn't even sure if an ambulance would come all the way out there.

I was having a hard time breathing, and my heart was racing and skipping the occasional beat. I was telling myself over and over that I wasn't having a heart attack because I'm too young, I had lost a lot of weight, I have low cholesterol, and I wasn't doing anything strenuous at the time of onset. But then the doubts started to creep in: women don't experience heart attack the way men do as the pain is often atypical; maybe I'd over stressed my heart being heavy for so long, and now was the time it was going to give out; we have a history of heart problems in the family, etc.

I decided to call my mom to see if she thought I should go to a hospital, or whether I should try and wait it out. (When you're in trouble, don't you always call your mom? Or someone else's mom even…?) While I was on the phone trying to wheeze out what was happening to me, I was hit with a wave of pain that doubled me right over, and I dropped the phone. The pain caused me to let out a loud yell, and I could hear my mother on the phone hollering for me to pick it back up.

Unbeknownst to me, my husband's business partner, Mike, was outside unloading equipment into the storage barn, and he heard me yell. He came running in, asking what was the matter. I could barely squeak out words at this point, and given the fact that I survived a car accident that required six months of hospitalization and level one trauma care, I could not believe the pain I was having.

Mike grabbed the phone, and my mom told him to get me to a hospital. You have to remember that I'd had a few complications along the way, and only God knew what this was. So Mike threw my nightie-clad, barefoot self into the truck, and away we flew at about a million miles an hour to the closest emergency room.

The closest emergency room, by the way, is in a tiny little village in a hospital with six beds. Yup. Six beds. When I got married and moved out to the country, my husband told me that this was the closest hospital in case of an emergency. I told him in no uncertain terms that I'd literally have to be dying to go to that little tiny hospital. Be careful what you say….

We pulled up to the emergency entrance and were met by a doctor and a paramedic. They put me on a gurney and wheeled me into a curtained area that was literally three feet inside the door. No lie, the entire emergency room is smaller than my family room. They slapped oxygen and a pulse-ox monitor on me (pulse oximetry monitor — the clip thing they put on your finger), and tried to get me to tell them what was wrong.

I gasped out that I was in horrific pain, seven months post-gastric bypass surgery, related the minimal details of my car accident three years before, and told them I couldn't breathe and my heart was doing funky things. They kept telling me to breathe slowly and to calm down.

I was as calm as I could get given the circumstances, because I knew that if I was having a heart attack, there was a doctor, two paramedics, and three nurses there to deal with it. I was breathing as slowly as I could, but it was hard when I couldn't expand my chest to draw in air.

They listened to my heart and lungs, they took my blood pressure, they took blood, and they took x-rays. Finally, they gave me some pain meds and some muscle relaxers. About an hour or so later it subsided. I felt like somebody had beaten the living daylights out of me with a baseball bat.

My husband showed up somewhere in the middle of all this, just about the time they were telling me that it was probably just stress, and I'd probably had a panic attack or some other psychiatric event, because they couldn't find a thing wrong with me. To me, it sounded as though they were telling me that they thought I was imagining all this, but I'm sure that's not what they meant. They simply didn't have a definitive answer, and were looking for a likely or common cause. I can assure you, however, there was something terribly, physically wrong that day.

As a person who's suffered from Post-Traumatic Stress Disorder (PTSD) as a result of my car accident, I can tell you that I am acutely familiar with panic attacks, and this was not a panic attack. This was my chest being crushed in from all sides like I was in a giant vise grip. This was almost unfathomable pain. This was purely physical in nature and had nothing to do with stress, or panic attacks, or PTSD, or anything. This was not something I wanted to experience again.

I stayed in bed the next day because I was so incredibly sore. The following day I went back to work, and told our nurse friend Judy about the ordeal. She told me that if it ever happened again to go to a bigger hospital as soon as it started, as they might be more familiar with this type of problem. She wasn't sure what it was either, but she said if it was muscle cramping, that the heart is a muscle too, and I should take it very seriously. At least she confirmed that I wasn't crazy (well, not about this anyway...).

I've had the experience several times since then, and each time I immediately headed it off with prescribed muscle relaxers and pain meds. Karen, and several others we've spoken to, have since experienced this type of scramp as well. Judy (our nurse friend), says that she has encountered patients in the ER who've lost large amounts of weight, and present with the same symptoms. Yet still, the question looms: "Why is this happening, and what causes it?" Which brings us to a conversation we had with our friend, Mark, a massage therapist.

Mark is the head of a therapeutic massage program at a local college, and he theorizes that toning exercises and massages every couple of days (even self-massages) might help prevent this experience in the legs and torso by keeping the muscles and fascia loose — a technique called myofascial release. Preventing dehydration also seems to help, as does keeping up your potassium (eat those bananas) and magnesium levels, and being vigilant about taking your vitamins.

What medical literature we have found refers to this pain as myofascial pain ("myo" meaning muscle, and "fascia" meaning the tissue covering the muscle). We've found documented evidence of other people presenting in an ER with exactly the same symptoms thinking they were having a heart attack. It turns out there were no heart attacks, simply the myofascial pain. No notation was made regarding whether or not any of the patients had lost large amounts of weight prior to onset.

Dr. Baker has continued to research this type of scramp, and tells us that this phenomenon is most likely from calcium or magnesium shifts associated with weight loss. Spasms are the final result, can be significant (understatement of the century here!), and are most often noticed in the legs and at the lower end of the rib-cage. The roles calcium and magnesium play in the process of weight loss are not yet fully understood, nor are the roles played by the substances affected by calcium and magnesium well understood in situations involving losses of significant amounts of weight. At this time it is unproven as to whether it is related to too much, or not enough calcium in the body. Interestingly though, calcium is extremely important for the proper functioning of muscle, specifically for a muscle's ability to contract.

No matter the causative theory, if you experience one of these scramps, putting a heating pad on the area seems to help somewhat, also alternating ice and heat may help. It has been our experience that laying on your left side helps with your heart pounding, and giving in to the need or reaction to stretch your torso only leads to doubling the pain. We've both found that allowing your body to curl up is preferable to trying to lay out straight as far as pain levels go. Sitting up may worsen the pain as well, as your torso seems to want to try and compact together. We also suggest drinking water in small sips, and drinking as much as possible.

Probably the most important thing, however, is to remain calm. Force yourself to calm down, relax your muscles, and breathe as slowly and deeply as possible. If you are alone when a scramp strikes, make sure you alert someone else of the situation. If others in the house are sleeping, wake someone up. Just knowing that you're not completely alone seems to help with relaxing and calming yourself. If the pain becomes too much, or you are experiencing an inability to breathe or your heart is beating erratically (not just fast), seek immediate medical attention. Better safe than sorry.

Knowing what you're going through, and not assuming that you're just stressed, or having a panic attack, will be helpful as well. If you seek medical attention, be sure to inform the doctors that you are a weight loss surgery patient, and explain in detail what you are experiencing. If you're experiencing a torso scramp, don't be at all surprised if they examine you to rule out a heart attack. Let them make sure everything is working properly, and let the safety of being with trained medical professionals who can help you in any situation assist you in trying to relax and breathe.

Just knowing that this could happen is probably one of the best pieces of information you'll get out of this book. Glad we could suffer, so you don't have to. Julie and Karen's Prognosis: This ranks ten out of ten Ow-ies! on the Ow-ie! Meter, but will probably not adversely affect your life expectancy.

And last, but by no means least, are our favorite after-effects of all time.
Drum roll please…. (Read the next two chapters!)

Chapter Five

➤ A U T O   E J E C T ➤

Julie M. Janeway
Karen J. Sparks

This short, but oh so very important chapter is dedicated to the phenomenon of "dumping." For anyone who has experienced dumping syndrome, it comes as no surprise that it is being afforded its own chapter.

"Dumping syndrome" is something that occurs in gastric bypass patients as a result of the body's inability to absorb and process certain types of foods, or because food moves too quickly through the digestive tract. "Rapid gastric emptying" or "dumping syndrome" occurs when the small bowel fills too quickly with undigested food from the stomach.[1]

The entrance of the food material causes fluids to shift from other tissues into the intestine via osmosis. The increased fluid volume causes a rhythmic contraction that pushes food through the intestine (peristalsis), and consequently causes diarrhea. The loss of fluid from the capillaries can cause decreased blood pressure (hypotension), which may result in weakness, dizziness, and a rapid heartbeat.[2]

"Early" dumping begins during, or right after a meal. Symptoms of early dumping include nausea, vomiting, bloating, diarrhea, abdominal pain or cramps, feeling flushed, sweating, dizziness, weakness, rapid heartbeat, and/or shortness of breath.[3]

"Late" dumping happens one to three hours after eating. Symptoms of late dumping include weakness, sweating, dizziness, and abdominal pain or cramps.[4] Many people have one or both types, and most people have their own unique combinations of symptoms.

Make no mistake, however, if you have dumping going on, you know about it. There's no confusing it with anything else. When you're experiencing dumping, you are both afraid you're going to die, and afraid you won't.

Dumping syndrome occurs in most gastric bypass patients, although some people claim never to have experienced it (we think they lie...). It's a safe bet to assume that if you have gastric bypass surgery, you will experience this thrill ride. Six Flags®, Disney World®, and the ninth ring of hell have nothing on dumping!!

If you're reading this book as a resource in helping you make a decision whether to have surgery, you also need to understand that this phenomenon doesn't happen every time you eat. In fact, you quickly learn through the theory of negative conditioning to FOREVER avoid whatever caused it to happen in the first place!

The usual suspects include grease, sugar, rich foods like ice cream, high carbohydrate foods, eating too fast, not chewing well enough, and dehydration. Good bariatric centers will tell patients to stay away from eating sugary, greasy, rich carbohydrate filled foods. The staff members at MMPC® in fact gave us these warnings on several occasions. As we stated earlier in this book, I tend to be a person who has to test the limits to see if they really apply to me. Yes, I was the kid who had to stick her hand on the burner to determine whether or not it was really hot.

I will now relate to you the truth about Pop-Tarts®. The truth about Pop-Tarts® is that they are in fact filled with as much sugar as the box says. I thought that maybe I could just eat half of a blueberry Pop-Tart®, and maybe if I left off the dry outer edges, it would be okay. I drastically miscalculated, and promptly spent the next six or so hours looking and feeling like a heroin addict spending her first night in detox.

To make matters worse, the phone rang while I was begging for death, and it was Karen. She could tell that I was in some sort of distress by the ghoulish way I answered the phone, and she of course immediately inquired what was wrong. When I croaked out, "I ate half a Pop-Tart®," I expected to hear some words of concern and support. Instead she quickly said she'd call me back later. Apparently, she had to get off the phone because she was spontaneously combusting with laughter on the other end of the line.

Karen did call back later (about seven hours later...) when she could finally get in enough air to form a complete sentence without busting a gut laughing. She matter-of-factly (and just a little self-righteously) told me that Dr. Baker told me not to do that. I said, "I know." She then asked me why I ate the Pop-Tart®. I said, "Well, I only ate half, and I only ate the middle." She roared laughing again, and said she'd call me back. To this day we can't walk down the Pop-Tart® aisle in the grocery store without her having a laughing fit. So, the purpose of this story is to demonstrate that the doctors and scientists have proven that sugar will cause gastric bypass patients to keel over and pray for death.

Now my stories about food limitations don't end there. I have stories about bagels, rice, birthday cake, and ice cream too. Suffice it to say, if my having to eat ice cream would create world peace, and allow me to buy and sell Bill Gates, I'd still have to think long and hard about it. By the way, because of dumping, we've conclusively proven that negative conditioning isn't just a theory. Scientists take note.

So, if panting like a dog, having your heart beat out of your chest like you're in mile 24 of a marathon, getting cramps that register on the Richter scale, having bed spins like you've been on a prom night bender, and experiencing the kind of nausea even astronauts don't get in the G-force simulator sounds like fun, then give us a call because the ice cream and Pop-Tarts® are on us.

Now I wouldn't, however, want to give you the impression that Karen is the rational compliant one in the group. In fact, I remember a little incident a couple months back in a restaurant just outside of Detroit. We were on a big shopping trip (translation: retail therapy), doing important woman business, don'tcha know. We stopped to get some dinner because we needed to keep up that protein intake. I ordered some type of chicken dish because I still don't do well digesting beef. Karen decided to order a hamburger, and she ordered it with double onions, despite a warning from me not to do that.

Onions for some reason are hard to digest when you eat them in larger chunks. They seem to be okay chopped into small pieces in things like salsa, but red onions seem to be especially bad. Of course, she ordered double red onions on her burger, even though Dr. Baker told us not to eat them.

Karen proceeded to ditch the bun, and she cut her hamburger and onions up into very small pieces that she ate slowly and chewed very well. She stopped when she was full, and like so many other restaurant meals, put the rest in a to-go box to be later delivered to the styrofoam jungle that is her home refrigerator.

We left the restaurant and got in her car. After all, we still had so much bargain hunting to do. But alas, poor Karen succumbed to the onions. We spent the better part of an hour stuck in the freezing cold in a mall parking lot while she turned shades of green that don't even appear in nature.

But Karen is a true fighter, and as soon as she could get her head off the dashboard, she summoned up the willpower to begin the hour and a half ride home. She wouldn't even hear of letting me drive home despite the fact that she now had her head stuck out the door auto ejecting at least some of the onions. So I buckled myself in, said a prayer, and quietly emptied out one of the bags from my shopping trip in case she didn't get the window open in time as we drove. (I just thought it prudent to attempt to prevent a potentially nasty stain that the dry cleaner might not want to touch.)

Due to multiple gas station restroom stops, it took over three hours to get home that night. Now Karen has an almost freakish phobia of onions. Another aisle in the grocery store that's off limits....

The reality is, everyone who has gastric bypass surgery will eat something, advertently or inadvertently, that will cause dumping. Some people can't tolerate chicken, or beef, or fish for the longest time. Karen couldn't tolerate garlic in any form or amount for almost eight months. With other people it's potatoes, or fruit. I couldn't tolerate anything that had carbs in it like bread or pasta or potatoes for almost a year. But it can be any kind of food, even if you think you're being careful.

I ate some southern fried chicken, minus the skin, and made myself gloriously sick one day. Thank God for napkins and bathrooms because what is auto ejecting from you isn't too picky about the exit path.

So what can you do to limit your interactions with what can only be likened to an infantile projectile vomiting-dysentery-nervous breakdown hybrid? Drink lots of water. There are so many reasons you should be drinking lots of water (see Chapter Eleven), not the least of which is to prevent dumping. Also, chew your food well, eat slowly, and follow the instructions regarding foods to avoid.

If you end up in a dumping syndrome situation, then we advise lying on your left side (bathroom floor optional), and taking small sips of room temperature water. The rest is just waiting it out and letting it pass. It might take a half hour, and it might take six hours. We suggest stashing a pillow and a blanket behind the toilet.

Also, I think I should make a point about other things you should avoid, like drinking alcohol. Although the alcohol didn't cause dumping (but it can), I think it's important to tell you why they warn you not to drink after gastric bypass.

Once again, I decided to test my personal physical limits and test Dr. Baker's authority. I was on vacation in Florida with my husband at an outdoor restaurant on the Fort Meyers Beach boardwalk. I ordered a banana daiquiri thinking, "How much alcohol can really be in a goofy umbrella drink like that anyway?" I took three small sips of my drink over about a five-minute time span. Two hours later, when I could finally focus my eyes, my husband peeled me out of my chair, aimed me at the car, poured me in, and took my liquified body back to the hotel.

Don't drink alcohol. You might as well be main-lining it like an addict. It goes right into your blood stream in full force; and I mean *right* into your blood stream. Three sips and I was sliding under the table, screaming at a barking dog passing by, and laughing like a hyena. So just a word of caution here: if after gastric bypass you want to slide under the table, or dance on one, at least you'll be a cheap date. But if you would like to keep your dignity and good reputation intact, refrain from drinking alcohol. Listen when they tell you to avoid things... save yourself the trouble.

Chapter Six

GETTING A
"BUILD-YOUR-OWN-CAT"
KIT

Karen J. Sparks
Julie M. Janeway

What did you say?... A cat with every surgery? What a deal! Or... not such a deal.... If you are a recipient of a "build-your-own-cat" kit, you can't give it back. Cat lover or not, you just have to deal with what you get. Another thing you need to understand is that your kit will arrive with little warning, and yes, unfortunately, some assembly is required.... Let me explain.

No matter what type of weight loss surgery you may undergo, they tell you there may be some hair loss due to the anesthesia, and the stress on the body. They also warn you that if you don't take in enough protein your hair may also become dry and brittle, and begin to thin. A few lost hairs? Okay, I can deal with that.

I knew that hair loss was a possibility, and thought I was prepared. (Silly me!) I have always had a more than generous head of hair, one thing that in my mind, being overweight didn't affect (my ears are rather cute too). How was I to know that for too long I'd been taking my tresses for granted? That was all about to change.

About four weeks into my recovery, I noticed my hairbrush becoming fuller and fuller. I called Julie and told her I was concerned about the amount of hair being collected in my brush, and if it didn't slow down soon, I would possibly be able to use all that hair to build my own cat! So began the days of my brush containing more hair than usual, and little did I know that the first shipment of my "build-your-own-cat" kit had arrived.

Here is where I feel I must clue you in as to my general attitude toward the feline homogeneous. As a rule, I have not always been that fond of kitties. As long as they belonged to someone else, life was good. Julie has two "cat-children," and next to God, I think they are the most important things in her life. (Husband ranks third?)

Conan O'Brien has a segment he produces on his show that pokes fun at what certain celebrities' children might look like if they should mate. Given Julie's genetically based, crazed love of cats, if Julie and Matt were to have a child, I swear it would be a cat! (I'll give you a moment to get that picture out of your head.) Needless to say, she's found more humor in the "build-your-own-cat" kit, than I have. Now that you have that background, let's move on.

At this point in my hair loss experience, I had not yet noticed any excess hair in the shower, but it has always been normal for me to see a little hair caught in the drain screen. Things were going along well — a little scrub here, a little lather there. Showers went on as usual. But then about six weeks post-surgery, the major shipment of my "build-your-own-cat" kit arrived. I was *SO* not prepared for that delivery.

I was getting ready for work one morning when "the kit" arrived. I had no idea that assembly of the "build-your-own-cat" kit would take place a handful at a time – or in my shower. As I ran my hands though my hair to rinse out the shampoo, I felt the loose hair caught in my fingers. Gently and fearfully pulling my hands down, I looked at them in sheer disbelief. Two tangled balls of soapy hair sat there looking back at me. Chills and nausea passed like a wave though my entire body. Looking down in the shower I realized that the fuzzy lump resembling a small, wet kitten hovering over the drain was actually a good portion of my own hair as well. I closed my eyes, and despite the water hitting me, I could feel the tears begin to slide down my face.

To tell you the truth, I was seriously scared. Scared of what was happening. Scared to look in the mirror. Scared of it getting worse. I was scared through and through. Each time I looked in the mirror in the days and weeks that followed, I began to see my brothers' receding hairlines. As I tried different ways of styling my hair to cover them up, I began to discover bald spots forming in different locations across my scalp. Would it stop? If so, when, and how?

When I took a shower I was very careful not to scrub my scalp too hard for fear of even more hair coming out. My anxiety over my hair completely disappearing doubled on a daily basis, and I began to consider what I might do. Cut my hair very, very short? Shave my head? Wear a hat? My mom suggested looking into the prospects of buying a wig. My mind worked overtime attempting to come up with a way to compensate for my hair becoming M.I.A. Dread, panic, and nausea aside, I simply wasn't going to let this beat me down.

Deciding what to do with my remaining three hairs was a dilemma. You should also know that the hair loss after-effect was not just mine. Julie experienced it as well. Julie possesses an excessively thick, full, and mostly uncontrollable, naturally curly Irish mane of dark hair – and it, too, was falling out.

Between Julie and her two cats, everywhere I sat at her house, I either had cat fur, or Julie hair on me. (I think the cats were having "sympathy" hair loss.) To a person who lives alone, and who is not used to having *any* pet hair on her clothes, even just a bit here and there was weird. In response to my whining about the cats shedding in sympathy with her, she told me that if I didn't want their hair (or hers) on my clothes to stay off the furniture! (She says that's why they call it "fur"niture.)

Anyway, we discussed our dilemma, considered our options, and determined we needed professional help before I went bald, the cats went bald, Julie went bald, or her husband Matt went missing under a pile of shed hair. So, I kidnapped Julie and off we went to see her hairstylist, Saul. Incidentally, you have to see a good and reputable hairstylist. Don't see the person at the $6, two-minute haircut store!! This is mega-important stuff. See someone with advanced training and education.

At the salon Saul was very kind and compassionate as Julie and I explained the dilemma with our hair. Although Julie's hair was thinning rapidly, I was in balding crisis, so we agreed on hair triage. I went first.

We began to tell Saul how this situation came about. You have to understand that at about six weeks post-surgery, it's still hard to tell people (strangers especially), that you've had weight loss surgery. You're still kind of sensitive about it. So, after relating that tidbit in hushed tones, we continued the story.

We told Saul how I was not exactly thrilled with the protein drink provided to me in those first few weeks, nor could I consume the required amounts. (They've since changed brands of protein drinks given to surgery patients.) I simply didn't want to eat anything at all, and my initial thoughts and reactions were, "Are you kidding me here?" I forced in as much as I could, thinking it would be enough. It was to my detriment that I didn't get enough protein in those early days following the surgery, and that is what prompted the hair loss. Saul listened with rapt attention.

Now, you must understand that your hair won't fall out just because you didn't eat enough protein the day before. This is a cumulative thing, and will take a few weeks to cause this kind of effect. Once you get that behind in your protein, however, you're forever playing catch-up to restore it. Don't put yourself in that situation.

I sense the panic as you read this, but not to worry. When I consulted Dr. Baker about my hair loss, he assured me my hair would restore itself. He told me just to keep up the good fight, maintain the all-critical protein, and things would work themselves out. I had trusted this man with my life; therefore, I believed I could trust him with my hair.

Saul nodded in complete understanding of the situation. We expressed our concerns that any sort of chemical application would cause more hair loss. We related our fears of coming in with a little hair left, and going out with none. We asked for help and guidance. Saul gave me a reassuring pat, Julie a confident look, and began to explain what needed to be done.

Hairstylists are licensed professionals in most states. If you ask for their guidance, they usually have the requisite expertise to deal with your hair-raising, hair loss predicament. Here are some of the tips our professional Aveda® hairstylist recommended.

Wash your hair every two or three days instead of every day. It doesn't need that kind of agitation. Also, coloring your hair helps to give it a fuller and thicker look because it actually expands the hair shaft. The addition of highlights and lowlights gives the illusion of fullness because it reflects more light. Add a nice cut and style (medium and shorter, but not short styles are better), and you are well on your way.

Your hair salon will probably recommend their product line as far as volumizing and thickening products. There are many excellent product lines in salons, including shampoos and conditioners, but beware the amount of styling product you use in your hair. If it weighs down the hair shaft, gravity will work against you by pulling the shaft out of the follicle, defeating your purpose. Nature based products (like those offered by Aveda®) are generally better than completely chemically contrived ones, but it becomes a personal choice.

The reality is, however, that salon products can get expensive (but if you use them correctly, they're generally comparable in the long run). Let's face it though; unless you have an unlimited amount of disposable income, the one-stop shopping center, health and beauty aisle is looking pretty good. (But remember, although salon products may be a little pricy, like you-know-who says: "I'm worth it.")

Many products are available in your local stores that will work for adding fullness and volume at a reasonable price, including remedies like Rogaine®. For those of you who may find yourselves in situations of severe hair loss, always consult a physician before self-medicating with any of the remedies such as Rogaine®, Minoxidil®, and such. Each experience is individual, and there may be other factors contributing to your particular hair loss episode.

Besides products that simply regrow hair, there are multitudes of volumizing, thickening, and shine inducing styling products available in stores. But, be careful with getting carried away on the volumizing products; more product does not necessarily mean more volume. It just might mean more scrubbing to get it out, and more related hair loss, so cut down on the abuse you're giving your hair.

Cutting down on the abuse also means reducing the amount of blow-drying (blow dry on low, at low heat, and use fingers not brushes), and limiting the use of curling and flat irons, especially. Also, the use of hair binding items such as hair clips, ponytail bands, and the like aren't good for thinning hair, as they tend to pull on the hair shaft, and/or break it off. Our hairstylist's advice: Be kind to your hair, it's injured.

Of course, being kind to your hair necessitates following the post weight loss rules, a message we've resonated throughout this book. Drink plenty of water to keep yourself hydrated, take your prescribed vitamins every day, and eat what you are supposed to in order to keep up with that all important protein quest.

Protein intake is critical not only to your overall system, but especially to your hair, which consists primarily of keratin, a type of protein. When your body is deficient in a nutrient such as protein, it begins a process of shutting down the least necessary assets, much like the electrical breakers in your house shutting down one outlet before the whole system blows out. This is why your hair falls out if your protein intake is too low for too long. Your system has shut down shipping protein to the hair, in order to continue supplying other vital systems instead. Keeping up the protein supply is the real trick.

After you have had your weight loss surgery, the hardest thing is actually learning to eat again (see Chapter Twelve). I am here to tell you that most likely you won't want to eat, but you must. It's hard, but if you like your hair just the way it is – EAT! (or drink, as the case may be…) Protein and vitamins are critical. Fact stated. Tattoo it on your forehead for future reference.

What you should also note for later reference is that if you lose your hair, you should choose to look at it as an opportunity for your first makeover (guys, this means you too). Time to update that look!

Despite the fact that I am considered a highly educated person, my sense of style and skills in promoting my own self-image were minimal at best. Being overweight for the entirety of my life, I would not engage in anything that would draw attention to myself. Hair and make-up? Why? I mean, I'm trying to hide in plain sight here!!! Why would I draw attention to myself? Geez…!!

Once you decide to have weight loss surgery, however, or if you have begun your journey already, you will start to discover another physical person emerging out of that old physical you. For me, it just so happened that she began to emerge with less hair…but emerging she was.

Because I've never been one who was concerned much with my outer presence (other than being clean and tidy), when Julie suggested we visit the stylist at her Aveda® "day-spa" to deal with the hair loss issue, I was pretty concerned that I was in a little over my head. But I trust Julie like a sister; I thought about it, and as I said, I kidnapped her from her house one day, and away we went.

When Saul suggested coloring my hair, I was a bit reticent as I've never colored my hair (gray or no gray). But since Julie has always been a hair and make-up diva, I figured I had no choice but to trust her and Saul when they told me that was what I needed. (Incidentally, Julie took away my car keys so I couldn't leave.)

Once I made that decision, I thought, "What the heck, you might as well do whatever else you think is necessary while you're at it." The two of them looked at each other with evil little grins on their faces (too evil for my liking), and they assured me that this makeover was going to help my hair loss problem, and make me feel like a whole new woman. After all, wasn't that the point of having the surgery? To become a whole new woman? They saw that my defenses were down, and they went in for the kill.

My hair loss misfortune inadvertently turned into one of the most fortunate experiences since my surgery – a serious "little victory." My hairstyle really hadn't been updated in years, and the new one brought out my features and made my face look thinner. (Yeah!) My new color and highlights worked so much better with my skin tone that it made me look younger. (Yeah!) I just couldn't believe it was me.

Saul taught me to style my hair with minimal effort, and I learned all about what was good for it, and what wasn't. Then they took me to see the make-up artist. Being an artist myself, I can appreciate the talent it takes to draw the human face, but I've never been able to draw worth anything when it came to drawing *on* my own face. I just knew that I'd end up looking like a recent graduate of clown-college, but I figured I could always go and wash it off.

Julie, recognizing my trepidation (maybe the death grip on the chair gave me away?) told the make-up artist that I'd never worn make-up, and to do something extremely natural and light. She also told her to explain to me what each product was, what it was for, and to write down the order in which they were applied. I closed my eyes, and slumped back in sheer resignation to what I was sure would be my utter humiliation in looking like a carnival freak.

I was determined not to look as she was applying the products, and I was only listening half-heartedly to what she was saying, but curiosity got the better of me once or twice, and I peeked. What I saw when I peeked wasn't so bad, and then I thought, "The worst is yet to come." But it never did.

When she was finally finished, I took a deep breath, and squinted open one eye. I was indeed shocked at what I saw. What I saw was me – only better. She had done exactly what Julie suggested: a light and natural look that just enhanced my own features. I was amazed. I had eyelashes!! My eyebrows had shape!! I was astounded, and very, very pleased. Thinking back, I don't know why I ever thought that a trained make-up artist, or Julie, would ever let me come out looking like a Jackson Pollack painting. Must have been the fear talking.

While Julie was getting her hair repaired, I must have spent at least an hour and half sitting there looking at myself in the mirror. Was that really me? Me, who came in all frazzled at my hair loss situation? Really? Is it possible that I came in one person, and am going out another? Is it really that easy? Yup!

With the help of a good hair stylist, a little color, an appropriate hairstyle, and products to promote fullness, you can get past the hair loss issue in grand fashion. My hair has come back in good order, and the world still turns. You may think your surgeon is a miracle worker for helping you through this life saving surgery, but in a hair loss crisis, a good hair stylist and an accompanying friend are worth their weight in gold.

Although a full makeover is not really part of dealing with hair loss, you should do it anyway. I used to say, "Hair and make-up? Why?" Now I say, "Hair and make-up? Why? Because the new you deserves it, that's why!

As Julie and I have stated throughout this book (and we'll say it again to anyone who'll listen), whatever comes your way, whatever the after-effect with which you must deal, do what you have to do, and move forward. Deal with it as best you can, and find the solution that works for you.

Hair loss doesn't have to happen to you, because as we've said it is almost totally preventable. Even if you don't have any hair loss issues, you should still consider going to see a good stylist anyway, just to update your look. By six weeks post-surgery, you'll really be starting to see the new you emerge. Give that new person a boost in the right direction, and remember: only your hairdresser really knows for sure....

Chapter Seven

THE SHADOWS OF
⟶ MY FORMER ⟵
SELF

Scott H. Glass, M.S., M.A., L.L.P.

In this chapter we get down to serious business – no tiptoeing around. You have two main reasons not to take bariatric surgery lightly: your surgeon will be going beneath the surface of your skin to do some serious rearranging of your intestinal tract, and you will be going beneath the surface of your psyche to operate on the shadowy memories, thoughts, and feelings that have gone unaddressed to this point. The latter deals with what's preventing you from losing the weight and keeping it off, and that is the focus of this chapter. It's not a really fun chapter, but it is an important and thought-provoking one, so hang in there with me for your own good, okay? Let's get started.

Have you ever heard the saying, "You reap what you sow?" A farmer who works hard to sow a crop will reap the reward of a good harvest. If he does not work diligently to sow and maintain a good crop, he will not get as good a harvest. The reality for you is that you, too, have reaped what you have sown. Recognizing that family history and genetics have influence as well, your obesity is a result of the choices you have made in your life. You have chosen to take in more calories than your body requires, and you have chosen to engage in more sedentary activities. These were your choices, and now you are reaping what you have sown.

I have heard time and again from bariatric surgical patients that "I have had to work hard to stay this heavy." "Obesity is what I get for living foolishly." "No one forced me at gunpoint to eat that food. I chose to eat it all by myself." "At the end of the day, I chose not to go for a walk; instead I chose to watch television." Choices always have consequences. Sooner or later, everyone will reap what they have sown.

I just met with a woman today who admitted, "It was just always easier and more fun to eat." Now, well over 100 pounds overweight, and with increasing and serious medical concerns, she experiences the cost of living in this manner. If she wishes to reap a different crop from what she has sown, she will have to change her mindset, behaviors and really examine what she values in life.

As a culture, we value comfort. We believe we are entitled to live a comfortable life. We believe we have the right to do things that make us comfortable. After a hard day at work, we believe we deserve to take it easy. We deserve a mixed drink when we are stressed or worried. If we don't feel like cooking, we are entitled to go out to eat. As a very obese society, we have based our lifestyles and behaviors on these perceived rights and entitlements, and consequently we have reaped what we have sown.

My point is not whether you do or do not have these rights. My point is that based on these ideas, your behavior has gotten you into serious health trouble. As long as you rely on these rights and entitlements, you will not overcome your weight problem. You have other rights and entitlements to rely on, however, like the right to a healthy life and a healthy body, being entitled to engage in activities of your own choosing, to eat healthy and nutritious foods, and to make choices because they are good for you, not just popular, easy, or expected. Shift the paradigm!

Recently, the discussion in a support group centered on eating during the holidays. The attitude of the group was one of defeat. "We can't change." "Holidays only come around once in a while." "We always host the meal at our house, so I have to do the cooking." "It's tradition. People are coming in from out of town, and they will be disappointed if I don't fix their favorites. They always look forward to my cookies."

Again, I am not saying you cannot or should not do these things. What I am saying is that by continuing to hold to these preset notions and the fear of change, you lock yourself into the same behaviors that got you in trouble in the first place. Value the companionship, the family, the memories, and the experiences. Do not value the food and the obligation to maintain unhealthy behaviors. Find alternatives that can be palatable to the majority of those involved. (You can't please all of the people all of the time....) Call it progress. Call it expansion. Call it creating new traditions. Call it whatever you want, but change the reality and be prepared for somebody to be resistant to how the changes will affect their lives – after all, you were.

It is a blunt fact that people want to live their lives the way they want to live them. We do not like to be told how to live our lives. How many times over the years have your doctor or loved ones encouraged you to lose weight, to change your eating pattern, or to start exercising? Granted, these changes are difficult, but did you work at it? Were you committed to the point of doing whatever it took to meet your goal? Did you change your thinking, your viewpoints, and your outlook? Maybe, but you certainly didn't make it a pemanent change or you wouldn't be reading this book.

Take exercise for example. People will say they do not have time to exercise. Many become angry or offended when encouraged to cut back in one area of their life to make time for exercise. They maintain there just isn't time. When encouraged to get up earlier in the morning to exercise, they respond: "Oh, I am not a morning person. I could never do that." When asked, if they could go to bed a little earlier so you wouldn't be as tired in the morning, they respond, "No, I like to watch the 11:00 news and a little bit of Jay Leno," or "I just don't have time with my stressful job and busy family." People are by nature incredibly resistant to change, especially when it is perceived as "drastic" change.

Change is not easy, but the fact is that if you continue your current style of living your weight and health will get worse, and your quality of living will decrease further. Ask yourself: "Is my goal to be comfortable now, or healthy later?" Which do you value more? The answer to these questions will ultimately determine whether you should even consider weight loss surgery.

Successful weight management after bariatric surgery requires full commitment and perseverance. It is not easy. If it were, everyone would have done it and we wouldn't be writing this book! There is no cure for obesity, but, you can do it if you are serious, admit the problem, take responsibility for solving the problem, and totally commit to creating a permanent solution.

After admitting you have a problem, you must also define the problem. You might be surprised to learn that the problem is not your weight. No, really!! The excess weight is really just a symptom of a deeper problem. Turning toward food for comfort, relaxation, or just something to do is a symptom of underdeveloped, or ineffective coping skills. In today's stressful, busy lifestyles we could all use a few more coping skills!

I have said many times, one of the single best methods of managing your weight is to manage your stress and emotions effectively by developing your coping skills. Stress and emotions influence most people to overeat, and stress and emotions often keep people overeating until they are overweight or worse. So, until a person learns to manage their stress and emotion in a healthy and effective manner, that person will continue to struggle with their weight.

There is no way to just make stress and emotion completely go away. It's just life, and as we all know: life is not fair. Sorry to have to tell you this, but surgery or no surgery, you will continue to experience disappointment, failure, rejection, anger, and many other emotions. Although some of the stressors may be different, the existence of stress will remain. The trick is to learn to cope better (and don't kill the messenger!).

Coping more effectively is about breaking the less effective and often unhealthy patterns, and substituting new and healthier patterns in their place. Take, for example, a situation in which you experience frustration over something that did not work out the way you had planned. In the past, because there was nothing you could do to change the outcome, maybe you dealt with the frustration, anger, and disappointment by getting a bowl of ice cream to soothe those prickly feelings and make yourself feel better. This pattern of responding to negative emotions by using food as a salve has not really helped you feel better, only make you feel worse in the longrun.

A more healthy and effective method might be to first go for a walk, even a quick walk around the parking lot if you are at work, to let off the steam. Then, once you have cooled off, call a friend or co-worker and vent. Verbalizing problems and venting emotions through words really does help.

You could also just sit down, by yourself, and write out or diagram the problem from a couple of different perspectives. What are your options with that project now that the first run did not turn out as you had hoped? What are the pros and cons of each option? What did you learn from this project? How can you do it differently next time? Write down your plans for attempt number two, and know you've dealt with your emotions in a productive, positive, and non-destructive way.

When your emotions are getting the better of you, and you want to resort to your old behavior of throwing food at the problem, here is a little chart you can use to help you in coping with various emotional situations. Stick it to your refrigerator and look at it before getting a snack from now on. The following example is just to get you started. Substitute where necessary with ideas that are specific to you, such as adding to the list of emotions, sad, worried, afraid, guilty, ashamed, or hopeless.

HUNGER	EMOTIONS
When I am legitimately hungry, I will eat a small piece/portion of:	*If I am experiencing an emotion, I will not get anything to eat. Instead I will do the following:*
Yogurt Cottage cheese	When angry I will — clean the garage or closet.
Cheese stick Granola bar	When lonely I will — call/write a friend, ask someone to meet me for a walk.
Nuts Banana Raisins	When stressed I will — write in my journal, talk to a co-worker, soak in the bathtub.
Apple Peanut butter and low fat crackers	When bored I will — get out my To Do list and get on with it!
Protein bar Carrots Melon Sugar-free Jello® or pudding Hard boiled egg	When feeling guilty over eating something I shouldn't I will — remind myself to think in the big picture, get over it, remember I am human, and move forward!
OR I will drink a glass of water!	When I'm feeling defeated I will — get out my "before" picture and remember that I am in a better and healthier place than I was then.
	When I am feeling — I will

If, after trying some of these ideas, you realize a need for more help, do not procrastinate! Call a trusted friend or family member, or even a professional counselor or pastor. Dealing with emotions in an effective and positive way is extremely important to the success of your weight management program, whether or not you ever choose to have surgery.

If you do choose to have surgery, then developing good coping skills will help you head off problems relating emotion to food in the future. You'll have to make the drastic change of exchanging excessive eating for life participation and emotional confrontation, and all the stressors and emotions that entails. You'll have to eat right, eat less, and get moving. Well, you know what you need to do, so what keeps you from doing it? This is the $64,000 question! As you are able to identify the obstacles that interfere with what you know you should be doing, you are getting closer to the root of the problem.

Perhaps one of your obstacles to success centers on your expectations for weight loss. Think back to the expectations you had for every weight loss plan you've ever tried. Be honest with yourself. Did you have grand, high hopes of a miracle lurking in the back of your mind somewhere? Did you really hope or expect that it would somehow just melt away the fat while you slept? If you somehow harbored these kinds of expectations, then you'd better drag them out now and have a look at them before you decide on bariatric surgery.

What are your expectations for life after bariatric surgery? If you are hoping for the "extreme makeover" and "happily everafter," you will be sorely disappointed. If you get nothing else out of this book, understand that you will probably just end up looking like an average size person. And that is okay!! You do not need to have any-more drastic changes than bariatric surgery will already bring you in your physical appearance and your inner confidence and self-esteem. You do not need to completely become something you're not, nor *should* you become something you're not! After surgery, you should essentially remain the same person on the inside that you were before surgery.

You will bring all the same attitudes, perceptions, and hurts that you have now into your life after surgery. Do not expect the surgery to change anything but de-crease your weight. You can generally expect life to be pretty average, although easier and probably a little more happy. Your marital status, the quality of your close rela-tionships, your place in life will all be quite consistent with your life before surgery. As long as you are realistic about the outcome, are accepting of yourself, are healthier than before, and are committed to not going back to your old ways, then you're on the right track.

It's not enough just to tell yourself you're being realistic, and you're okay with whatever comes your way. Don't tell your doctor or your behaviorist what you think they want to hear just so you can forge ahead in the process. Most importantly, don't tell *yourself* what you want to hear, or you won't make it through the process with any real success.

The process includes really understanding why you failed before, and correcting those behaviors and ideas now. The process includes creating a realistic and detailed image in your head of what life and the end result will be after surgery (or any weight loss plan for that matter). Creating that realistic, detailed image in your head specifi-cally includes a realistic, detailed, long-term program for maintenance. The process doesn't come to a screeching stop the minute you drop the majority of your weight. Maintenance is incredibly important.

This process you are considering requires you to be accepting of your life as it is now, willing to change for the better, and to move forward into the future and not attempt to recapture days gone by. Can you truly accept the age you are now, and live a healthy and full life from this point forward? Can you regret missed opportunities and events from your past, but move forward with expectations of creating great new life memories to replace those things that were missed in the past? Can you truly accept your body type and that you will most likely not end up with the body of a college athlete? Can you accept that life will be the same, while at the same time different once you lose the weight?

These may all be factors you've not really considered indepth with all or many of your previous attempts at weight loss and modification of your behaviors. These may have been major reasons why you failed in the past. Others include being ready and willing to have patience with yourself, and being prepared to properly deal with setbacks, delays, and disruptions in your pre-conceived plan and timeline. Are you ready for these? Really? Are you truly prepared, and do you really understand that you will have to deal with some physical pain, some moments or periods of emotional defeat, substantial fear and anxiety, and potential feelings of regret when things don't go as you have them planned in your head? Think long and hard about these things.

You need to be comfortable with all this, and once you've really examined these issues and been honest with yourself in all the darkest corners of your mind, then, and only then, when you decide to go forward with surgery or another plan of attack, will you be truly ready to totally commit to change and a new and healthy lifestyle.

So, what does it mean to be totally committed? Total commitment is not based on emotions or feelings that change with the day. Total commitment is not based on the expectations or desires of others. If you choose surgery, it is your body that is going to be operated on. You are the one that must learn to be content with less, and with different food. Your significant other isn't the one going under the knife, facing potential surgical risks, or changing their style of living. They don't have to be totally committed.

Total commitment is not based on appearance, ability, or in any way comparing yourself with others. Total commitment is a decision to stick with something because you believe it is best, and because it is consistent with, and will enhance your personal values. Total commitment is sacrifice, going forward even though it may cost you something valuable because you believe so strongly in the end goal.

If you are of the mind that you will try the surgical route to weight loss to see if it works for you, and then, if it doesn't, simply resume life as normal, STOP! Don't proceed any further with your plan for surgery. You are setting yourself up for misery and failure. This trip cannot be purchased on a roundtrip ticket.

Hernando Cortez, a Spanish explorer, set sail for Mexico, which was at the time recently discovered. His mission was to establish a Spanish colony there. His men were grumbling and threatening to turn back because of the difficult conditions. When they arrived in on April 21, 1519, after the men had stepped on shore, Cortez set the ship on fire to prevent any thought of abandoning their new settlement. This is commitment. Despite what might lie ahead, Cortez and his men were going forward. There would be no turning back.

If anywhere in the dark shadows of your mind you are holding onto "safety" thoughts of being able to go back to your old way of doing things if you don't like doing the work necessary to get and keep the weight off, then consider Barry — learn from Barry's mistakes.

Barry was a morbidly obese man with a sedentary lifestyle, and he experienced a severe, nearly fatal heart attack at age 40. His doctor told him that he needed to make significant changes in his lifestyle to improve his health. He took his doctor's recommendations seriously. He stopped drinking alcohol, stopped smoking, started exercising, and even discontinued some of his friendships because of their unhealthy influence on him. He began working fewer hours to decrease his stress, and learned to relax. He maintained these changes for about two years.

But then when the coast seemed clear, and it was smooth sailing ahead, he gradually returned to his former lifestyle. In his mid-forties Barry developed a severe panic disorder and, for a time, was unable to come out of his bedroom. With intense counseling, he re-entered society again, gradually increased his activity, and rekindled relationships with family and friends.

His counselor and family worked with him to make drastic lifestyle changes. He enjoyed improved health and increased quality of life, but, again, he maintained these healthy lifestyle changes for only about two years. Why? He admitted that although he enjoyed the improved health, he did not enjoy the behaviors, or the style of living necessary to maintain his improved health. In both situations he became complacent and gradually returned to his former lifestyle patterns, thereby increasing his risk to repeat the cycle all over again.

Eventually, Barry again put on a significant amount of weight as a result of returning to these old behaviors. He was once again advised by his doctor to get his life and his health under control or he wouldn't make it out of his forties. Barry took the doctor very seriously, and sought yet another way to modify his lifestyle to do what he could to ensure a longer, healthier life. Barry decided to have weight loss surgery.

During Barry's behavioral assessment, it was observed and explained to him that even his near-death experience did not keep his attention very long. Barry finally admitted to himself that he would rather live his life in a manner that was easy and enjoyable, than to adhere to the less comfortable lifestyle recommendations that would result in health and longevity. He was referred to counseling to help him explore his thinking and expectations if he wanted to go forward with bariatric surgery.

Barry went to counseling, and fudged his way through by telling the counselor all he thought she wanted to hear. Her report was positive and declared Barry a good candidate for surgery from an emotional standpoint. He had the surgery, still thinking it would be the magic pill to end his obesity and related health torments. He made it through the surgery without complication, and began to see the weight drop off.

While he was losing the weight in the honeymoon period, it did in fact seem to be the magic pill. Barry never changed a single habit, however, and to this day, two years later, Barry has gained back all the weight, and then some, and his co-morbidities have all returned. Barry has made his decisions about what he values in life. How sad that his life will be so short.

So, what about you? What do you value? A healthy vital life in the long run with a few concessions and fewer beers and burgers, or all you can eat at the big food buffet of life? Remember: the buffet closes. It's not open forever, and you can only eat just so much before you die in the attempt.

Every bariatric patient desires to lose weight, but only committed persons are willing to make the difficult decisions. It takes hitting bottom and deciding to climb back up a different way than you came down to be successful. Successful weight loss requires more than desire. Desire alone produces nothing but frustration. Desire produces action only when combined with commitment.

So, are you ready to give up some things in order to gain others? Are you ready, willing, and able to accept help? Are you ready, willing, and able to follow directions from trained professionals prepared to guide you and care about your success? Are you ready to get rid of old habits forever? Are you ready to leave your uncomfortable "comfort zone?" Be honest, and when you come to an answer, then decide on your next course of action.

If your next course of action is bariatric surgery, then you will enjoy remarkable change with your weight and appearance, however, these external changes will not compare with the degree of change you will experience on the inside. It is in the shadows of our inner thoughts, feelings, and memories where fear, anger, and self-defeating thoughts hide.

The emotional world can be shadowy. Looking into the shadows can be intimidating, frightening, and overwhelming. It's hard to see anything clearly. Fear hides in the shadows. Pain hides in the shadows. This is the domain of unresolved feelings and emotions. All that hides in the shadows can rise up against you when least expected. Knowing this engenders fear and reticence. Part of your journey to weight loss success is about getting rid of the fear.

Now, before we delve into this, it is important to clarify that obesity is not caused solely from painful, unresolved emotions. Obesity is a complex disease with numerous factors contributing to it. Some are within your control, and others are not. So, given these parameters, it is important for you to accept and enjoy who you are, control what you can, and deal with anything else without food as a crutch.

It is also important, however, to be truthful with yourself. Self-righteousness, entitlement, justification, and denial, are at the opposite ends of the spectrum from truth. To the degree we make excuses, or justify, or minimize why we continue our unhealthy patterns, we are in denial, and denial is the opposite of truth. But, just because we deny a problem, or deny the importance or significance of the problem, does not mean there is no problem on which to work.

We all have tendencies toward denial. We all want to think well of ourselves and for others to think well of us as well. We don't like to admit that we over-ate just because we wanted to, or that we didn't walk today just because we indulged our laziness. Admitting this doesn't make us feel good about ourselves, and we fear others will judge and not accept or like us. It is a lot more comfortable for us to blame it on how we were parented or our busy schedules than it is to admit weakness in ourselves.

Inwardly, these types of rationalizations provide relief. They take the pressure off and help us save face, even with ourselves. This is an indication of faulty thinking and/or denial of what we are doing to ourselves. At a deeper level, these are value statements. We make time for what we value. This is true whether what you value is self-defeating or self-affirming. The evidence speaks for itself.

You may have heard that you can tell the values of a person by looking at their checkbook. People spend money on what they value most. The same is true with our time, especially when the patterns are evident. Some people value comfort, so they choose to spend their time doing comfortable things. Some like to work on antique cars, or any number of other hobbies, so they spend their discretionary time on those endeavors. When we want to spend more time on our indulgences we do, and then leave less time for other responsibilities such as exercise, sleep, and relationships.

Our self-defeating values truly are difficult tendencies to confess to ourselves, let alone others. Honesty, vulnerability, authenticity, and understanding your self are vital to resolving the underlying issues that currently influence you toward unhealthy behavior. Facing the truth about yourself will result in healing from painful memories and emotions, followed by improved self-esteem. Further, as you address these unresolved emotional issues and begin to heal from them, your thoughts and feelings about yourself will improve, and your behaviors will follow suit.

Dealing with these raw emotions and hurtful memories is very difficult, I grant you. Making these changes is sometimes intimidating and overwhelming. This brings to mind one particular patient who became very upset when she learned that counseling would be necessary to decrease her symptoms of depression before moving forward with bariatric surgery. She explained that she had worked hard to bury her memories of abuse because of her weight, and that with counseling she would be required to dig them out and address them again. I had compassion for this woman. Her memories and experiences carried so much pain. It was more frightening to uncover them than to leave them buried.

So, why is it necessary to dig up these painful emotions? Why can't you just leave these memories safely tucked away in the shadows and get on with the surgery? This is a very good question. Unresolved issues like these can make us uncomfortable at best, and tormented at worst. We don't like thinking about them because they are too painful. There is often a degree of hopelessness because you cannot change the past, so what good would it do to think about these painful emotions?

We try to avoid these memories as best we can by staying busy, anything to stay busy. Getting involved, perhaps too involved, in relationships is a very effective means keeping the past in the past. Our efforts to anesthetize our painful emotions can propel us toward food. Certain foods taste good to us. Their texture and aroma are pleasing to us, and they are indeed comforting to swallow and have sit in our stomachs for a while. Eating is also very effective in helping you to "swallow" your pain and tears.

Perhaps you haven't thought about your painful or difficult memories in a long time, and you are not conscious of them presently, but they are contributing to your deeper feelings of discontentment, low self-worth, and consequential eating patterns. You may not be able to put your finger on it, but for some reason you need comfort, and food is a most convenient and readily available source. The fact that food is a comfort for you implies that there must be something in your life making you feel uncomfortable. Generally speaking, if there is no current source of discomfort in your life, then the source must be in the past or future.

If the source is in the past, you may be experiencing a degree of depression. If the source is something in the future, you may be experiencing a degree of anxiety. In either case, you will need to address this source of depression or anxiety to successfully manage your tendencies toward emotional eating and maintaining the bond between food and external issues.

To the degree that you turn to food for reasons other than physiological, you are putting food into your mouth for more subtle reasons such as cultural, emotional, or environmental. You may eat to give you something to do when you are bored, for companionship when you are lonely, relaxation when you are stressed and overwhelmed, comfort when you are angry, relief when you are hurting or experiencing guilt, or as a pick-me-up when tired, discouraged, or depressed.

Sit down with a pencil and piece of paper and ask yourself "Why do I often feel discontent?" "Why do I need to be comforted?" or "What do I need to be comforted from?" This is an interesting exercise to help you start looking into the shadows at the things that help to keep you overweight.

It is important, however, to shine some light into these shadows. It's not healthy to ignore or pretend that your life prior to bariatric surgery didn't exist. It did, and you have to reconcile those emotions. Although you think you have buried or wiped away all that hurt, pain, loneliness, and grief associated with the abuse, disappointment, shame, guilt, and fear of your life as a severely overweight individual, you haven't.

You can ignore it, you can pretend it isn't there, but it is there, and it will continue to adversely affect your decisions and patterns of behavior until you explore it and resolve it for good. Memories and feelings don't go away, but dealing with them effectively changes the links to current emotions, and changes the locus of control these memories and feelings have over your current situation. In the subconscious mind they have control. When brought to the conscious mind they can be controlled.

If you choose to have surgery, you'll undergo a metamorphosis of mind and body that will bring out a more healthy and complete you. This means you'll need to introduce yourself to this newly emerging person and begin to build a relationship.

In discovering who you've grown into being, you should first identify all the parts of you that haven't changed. These are generally things like your morals, your core life values, your principles, who you love, and how much you love them. This will help to ground you, and then you can begin to explore what other things about you have grown, have emerged, or have been freed through this process.

Learning to understand more about your traits, wants, desires, and feelings will help you to become more accepting of yourself. Accepting yourself, with all your faults and strengths, is the key to maintaining your commitment to your new lifestyle and newly found health. Learning to understand your "precious pain" and not giving into it, is also extremely important.

"Precious pain" is a term used by therapists and counselors to describe the conditions in our lives that we won't leave behind, even though they're painful and destructive, because at least they're familiar, predictable, and less scary than finding out about the alternatives. We see this principle at work when people stay in abusive relationships. They stay not because they like the abuse, but because at least it's a known quantity. The alternative, finding out how to fabricate a whole new and different life, is so scary and overwhelming that it's just easier to stay in the abuse.

Sadly, there are a number of persons who have suffered significant trauma, or physical or sexual abuse in their earlier years. A very common source of comfort and control available to children and adolescents is food. As children or adolescents, many traumatized people turned to food to help cope with painful experiences. As long as the cognitive and emotional wounds are not addressed and healed, these wounds remain in the shadows, sometimes very quietly, but all the while subtly influencing your self-esteem, self-confidence, emotions, and relationships.

These unresolved emotional wounds can have a strong influence on how you use your free time, as well as your degree and type of social activity. If you want to change your behavior, it is imperative that you look at the thoughts and feelings that influence that behavior. Do not fear releasing the precious pain, whether from trauma, physical or sexual abuse, or from the verbal and societal abuse heaped on people who commit the transgression of carrying too much weight.

This last type of precious pain is something the vast majority of overweight people live with every day. The weight, and the circumstances and conditions that surround it and its attendant issues, permeate all aspects of their lives. Thinking about losing the weight and having to find out how to cope with all new situations that don't involve being rejected, being stereotyped, being ridiculed, and assumptions being made about intellect, strength, and character can be a pretty daunting and intimidating task. Patients tell me, "I just don't know how to be thin!" Maybe it's just easier to stay fat? Maybe that's at least safer? Maybe that's how it's really supposed to be? No! It's not!

Surround yourself with people and professionals who will fill in the gaps for you when your coping skills are stretched a little thin. Be prepared to let them help you. If you are deciding to have bariatric surgery you *must* deal with the shadows of your former self that lurk in your psyche. Whatever lurks in the shadows currently, will continue to lurk in the shadows later. If allowed to remain hiding in the shadows after your surgery, these issues will gradually undermine and sabotage your weight loss efforts and long-term success.

Controlling and dealing with your psychological scarring is an important issue, but it doesn't have to be fully completed prior to surgery. For most, the process is begun during the time of the behavioral assessment, and continues throughout the surgery and the following weight loss period. As things begin to change on the outside, you'll have to reorganize and accommodate the change on the inside as well. Julie and Karen are going to talk a little bit more about that in Chapter Nine. Learn to deal with food and pain in a new way.

Let humanity back in to fill the spots formerly held by food. Fill your life with people and experiences, and see food only as a means to keeping you alive and healthy, and maybe for a few pleasant sensations or memories. Mostly, you should remember to negatively associate food with your old life and living in the precious pain. Food kept you anchored there, so cut the line and leave it behind. Accept your new life and know that you are normal, you're good enough for anything and anybody, and you are worthy of a good and healthy life.

Many persons looking for effortless weight loss solutions look to bariatric surgery as being the pinnacle of an effortless cure for obesity. They hope that the surgery will quickly undo or correct the result of years of unhealthy living and give them a new lease on life. What's wrong with wanting more quality and more years in your life? Nothing! In fact, these are pretty normal and healthy life goals, and we all have them. The issue of how to get and maintain them is where problems occur. This is where the value of the "psychological evaluation," or as I prefer to call it, the "behavioral assessment," comes in.

The behavioral assessment is an integral part of a more comprehensive assessment, which also includes medical and surgical consultations. The term "behavioral" includes everything necessary to manage lifestyle. I like to compare it to pre-employment screening, or pre-marriage counseling. It's the "reality check" to help ensure that though your head might be in the clouds, both feet are still planted firmly on the ground. It's a way to see if this is going to be a good fit all the way around.

The term "behavioral" is an umbrella term that encompasses many different behaviors. Some of these behaviors are obvious, such as eating and exercise behaviors. That's nothing new. But, there are many other more subtle behaviors also under this behavioral umbrella. These include your thoughts, feelings, motives, ambitions, perceptions, attitudes, goals, beliefs, values, and priorities. The list goes on to include your ability to manage your stress, emotions, time management, sleep, leisure, relationships, boundaries, and more. All of these subtle behavioral issues will directly influence how consistent you will be with your eating and exercise behaviors. In turn, it is the consistency of your eating and exercise that will directly determine how successful you will be with your weight loss and maintenance.

We usually recommend that your spouse, significant other, or other person who will act as your primary support person accompany you to the behavioral assessment.

While we are certainly interested in finding out about *you* from you, your support person can often be more objective about some things, and therefore provide valuable insight and information.

It is also helpful for us to gain a sense of how supportive your support person is. It is not unheard of for a support person to intentionally or unintentionally undermine the patient's efforts to lose weight. There are a variety of causes for this. A partial list might include the support person's insecurity, control, jealousy, or the disruption to their comfort level. When we observe this, we can either delve into it during the behavioral assessment or make a referral to an outside counselor. These relationship issues are vitally important to address before you will effectively manage your weight long-term.

Your honesty and integrity throughout the entire assessment process are also essentially important. Many patients are on the verge of desperation to have the surgery and will do almost anything to have it. It is not at all uncommon for patients to minimize their concerns or deny them altogether out of fear they will be denied the surgery. The vast majority of the time, however, covering up their concerns in order to manipulate their way into surgery catches up with them later. They might have been able to squeak through the assessment, gain authorization for the surgery, and have the surgery, but just as they are about to breath a satisfying sigh of relief, they develop more behavioral problems, or the behavioral problems they covered up previously get worse. Consequently, they are unable to develop any consistency with the lifestyle recommendations and fail to lose the expected amount of weight.

So, although they feel like they won the prize and were able to get the surgery, when they have post-operative complications that won't resolve, or significant frustration because they did not lose the expected amount of weight, they are not exactly sure they really won anything.

We talk a lot about medical and surgical risks associated with bariatric surgery, but you also need to know that depression is a risk for post-operative bariatric patients. If a person has tendencies toward depression pre-op, there is a greater risk for more, not less, depression post-op. When it is revealed through the behavioral assessment process that patients are struggling with depression, we immediately refer them to counseling, and/or for medical treatment.

The length of counseling will vary from a few weeks to possibly a year or more depending on the severity of the concern. Hearing us say that counseling will be required before moving forward with surgery is very disappointing for patients to hear, especially when they are already depressed. But, we have had countless patients come back later to thank us for prompting them toward counseling, saying how beneficial their counseling was and that they would never have initiated it themselves. After sufficient progress has been made toward the counseling goals, the patient will then be back on track for surgery.

Whether or not counseling is required before surgery, support and insight are most definitely required after surgery. Given the degree and difficulty of change that is necessary, you will need help. Persons who kid themselves and try to accomplish this on their own, fizzle out despite their best intentions and will power, therefore, a social support network is critically important.

These major life changes are very difficult to maintain over time (remember Barry?). Most people have high motivation going into, and for a time after bariatric surgery, but when the "shine" wears off, and when difficult life circumstances appear, they begin to fizzle out despite the best of intentions. The reason for the dismal long-term weight loss success rate is due to the fact that these lifestyle recommendations are so difficult to maintain over time. Don't be fooled. The same holds true for bariatric surgery patients. You need the loving support and encouragement from those persons in your life who care about you to remain diligent with the eating and exercise plans.

Don't try to go it alone. Social support begins with your family, your spouse, or significant other. They are the ones who know you the best, love you the most, and will be with you through it all. No one wants you to be successful more than those few close persons who love and respect you the most. They are the ones who know you privately. You can fool your co-workers, you can choose to tell your extended family half-truths, but your family, significant other, or spouse knows the whole truth about you. So, include them right from the get-go. From collecting information and learning about the surgery, making the decision to have the surgery, selecting a surgeon, and when to actually make the phone call to schedule your first appointment, include those people who will be your support network. Be sure to include a support person in all the pre-operative assessments. The more your support group knows about the process, the better they will be able to empathize and help you through the process.

After surgery, ask a few of them to call you once in a while to ask how you are doing with specific behaviors with which you know you will have trouble. Throughout this process, you will need a couple of people who care enough about you that when they call and you tell them you have not walked in a few days, they will come over to your house with their walking shoes on and say, "Get up, we're going for a walk."

Gently caution these loved ones, though, that you do not need them to be the food and exercise police. You do not need to be judged for not measuring up or meeting the goal for that day or week. You do not need negative or critical remarks. You do not need sarcastic sighs or facial expressions. There is a fine line between loving encouragement and legalistic monitoring. Loving accountability might be stern, and legalistic condemnation might be given with a smile, but you will still be able to sense the difference.

Another way to surround yourself with support is to commit to consistent participation in a support group. Meeting regularly with others who have gone through the same experience reminds you that you are not alone. Some in the group will be further along and will be able to coach you. On the other hand, you will be further along than some, so take the time to coach someone else. You will personally benefit as you encourage and coach them. Sharing in the success of others will encourage them and motivate you. Sharing in the weaknesses and failures of others will encourage them, while at the same time inspire you. In either case, it will be a win-win situation for you and other group members.

It has been our experience that persons who attend a weight loss support group manage their weight better than those who do not attend a weight loss support group. But, wait! It gets better! We've noted that persons who attend a weight loss support group frequently, lose more weight and maintain their weight loss better than persons who attend less frequently. Our results have shown there is a direct correlation between participation in a weight loss support group and successful weight management! You will experience not only more personal success, but at the same time, you will also be helping others succeed with their weight loss goals.

Your weight loss goals are perfectly attainable as long as they remain realistic, you explore what's hidden in the shadows of your mind, you modify those behaviors and underlying motivators, you do the work, and stay committed. Always remember that your multidisciplinary team is there to help you through whatever comes up, and you should not hesitate to ask for help from them, from family, friends, outside counselors, and even religious leaders. There's more support out there than you really imagined to help you deal with the shadows of your former self, and help bring you out of the dark and into the light of your new and vibrant life. Don't be afraid of the dark. Strike the match.

Flowers grow out of dark moments.

CORITA KENT

Chapter Eight

━ L I T T L E   V I C T O R I E S ━

Karen J. Sparks
Julie M. Janeway

I specifically wanted to write this chapter because it is very near and dear to my heart. It deals with many of the little things that mean so much to overweight people — things others so easily take for granted. It deals with fear and conquering fear. It deals with balance and perspective. It deals with joy and rebirth. It deals with struggle and perseverance. But most importantly, it deals with triumph.

As I struggled with making the decision whether or not to have this surgery, all the pain and fears of my life stood there plotting to wrestle me for control of the decision – I just didn't think I could take one more disappointment or failure. Among that unruly lot of pain and fears lurked a tremendous dread of undergoing surgery, because I had never experienced that type of thing. I was very scared of possibly dying on the table, as all surgeries that involve general anesthesia have a risk of death (although usually quite low). I was also very frightened that if I died, I would not have a chance to "fix" any of the things in my life that were messed up or delayed because of my weight and the related limitations. What to do? What to do?

In struggling with my fear of the surgical portion of the decision, I attempted to rationalize the facts. I am lucky that I come from healthy Scottish-Irish ancestry. Outside of the normal childhood illnesses, having babies, mom's gallbladder surgery, dad finding out he was allergic to penicillin, one broken arm, and a few emergency room stitches here and there, we are a healthy lot. Being a healthy person (no co-morbitities, although I was on the edge) rationally meant there was no reason to believe that I wouldn't come out of the surgery just fine and dandy. That being said, surgery still scared the beejeezies out of me!

My search for a final decision lead me to Dr. Baker's door. As I worked through building up my courage just to attend the orientation session, Julie shared with me the advice her sister had given her, "You can do anything afraid that you can do unafraid." I can't tell you how important that was to me. It carried me through the fear and uncertainty of making the decision, right up to being wheeled through the operating room doors, and beyond.

The "beyond" included a substantial fear of losing the weight. Who would I be? How would I look? Would I even know how to be thin? I've never been "not fat" before; will I know how to do it? Can I keep it off? Will it come back no matter what I do? It also included a substantial fear that if I actually lost the weight, would I be able to "get back?"

Would I be able to "get back" to being able to do things that I had once done? Would I be able to "get back" to doing things I'd only done for a brief time in my life? Would I be able to "get back" some of the lost opportunities in my life? Would I be able to "get back" on track with the life plans I'd laid out so long ago?

There were also many things I had spent a lifetime only being able to wish I could do, or didn't think I would ever be able to do. Would I be able to "get back" to a point where I could do them? Would I "get back" the courage to do them? This fear of the unknown gnawed ravenously at what resolve I'd managed to gather.

My resolve was further tested by my awareness that the majority of my weight would take a year or more to come off. As you begin this journey, or you are deciding if it is right for you, a year sounds like a long time. Let's face it: in the past when we thought of losing weight and going on diets, just the thought of how long it would take to lose a pound or two would derail our efforts. So yes, a year seemed like an eternity.

Yet, in some ways it didn't sound long enough to make the kind of changes you know will have to be made. But, in the grand scheme of things, I'd spent this many years living with the pain and limitations of my weight, so what was another year; and what was the difference between another year of the old pain and limitations, or a different set of anxieties? I made the decision, closed my eyes, and prayed for guidance and strength.

Following my surgery, the anxiety shifted to the "waiting." I thought, "Okay, I'm past the hard part, now I wait to see what happens." I waited impatiently to see, to feel, to experience whatever would present itself next. I waited to see if, and what I would "get back." My impatience was quickly rewarded, and the things for which I had waited became a series of events I named my "little victories."

Little victories for me were, and still are, little events that just seem to tug at my emotions as they happen. Little victories are the wound healers in your life. For every emotional memory of something bad that happened in your life as the result of your weight, a little victory makes it all okay; it tells you that it won't happen again. They are the emotional stabilizers you need as you deal with becoming a new person, in dealing with plateaus, body shape issues, and the other issues we'll talk about in the next chapter. Little victories are the happy milemarkers that let you know you are succeeding in your journey towards a new you.

What is truly and amazingly unique about each of your little victories is that they never go away, and they're as wonderful the first time you experience them as the hundredth. They impact you in such a way that you never forget the moment you first realized it was happening.

For those of you who can, you remember where you were when you heard President Kennedy had been shot. That day and that moment is indelibly etched in your mind; so too with your personal little victories. They become embroidered on your heart.

I remember fondly the day I first was able to buy a suit all in the same size. I'd never been able to do that before in my whole life. I remember with gratitude the day I got rid of the seatbelt extender in my car. I remember affectionately the day that Julie and I stood in a mall parking lot laughing about the skinny shadows we now cast. I remember vividly the first time after my surgery that I sat in a booth at a restaurant, and found out that I fit. That was an amazing day. I was so overcome with emotion, we sat there for almost an hour before I could concentrate enough to order something.

I happily remember all my little victories, and every time I re-experience them it's like the first time all over again. Every time I walk through the door of my pop-up camper and don't touch the sides, I giggle. Every time I cross my legs and they stay there, I smile and enjoy it all over again. For every bad memory that comes flooding back, or every old wound that re-opens while you're losing the weight, a little victory sneaks in and saps all its power away. They are the steps you take forward to a new life and a new attitude. They are also the wonderful steps you take in "getting back."

Incidentally, you should remember that not all things are really as worth "getting back" to as you might have thought. I "got back" to playing softball. I went and played a whole game, which was truly wonderful to do. I had a blast seeing my old friends, and reliving a snippet of my misspent youth. I also came home with a bruise on my shin where I got nailed with a wicked line drive, and aching muscles I didn't even know I had!

The bruise stayed for a month and half to remind me that I'd "been back," and to reassess whether or not I should ever "go back" again. Little victories help you figure out who you've been, who you were before surgery, who you are now, and who you're going to be. They're not just the milemarkers on the journey, they're the directional signposts as well helping you to determine your future paths, and which paths from your past are worth taking or not worth taking for a visit.

Although little victories can't necessarily give you back missed opportunities from your past, they may afford you replacement opportunities instead. Like many of you, I never had the opportunity to attend my senior prom. I always got to watch my sister get dressed up, be picked up by her date, and go to such events. Will my little victories provide me with an opportunity to go back and attend my senior prom? No, of course not. In fact, now I think the term "senior prom" pretty much means a dance for people 50 and older!!

But what I can do, and what I'm looking forward to doing, is attending my 30th class reunion knowing that I'll look better than I ever have, and enjoying my conversations and time with my former classmates, rather than having it all overshadowed by the specter of my painful high school years.

Little victories give you perspective. They help you to reframe what you want into things that are realistic and do-able, like having a great time at the reunion instead of wallowing in the pain of missed high school proms and dances. Little victories help you to see what's possible and practical now, rather than what you thought you might have wanted all along (like watching my friends play softball, not necessarily having to play softball). They help you to find your inner strength, and give you the patience to wait for the next one (which comes in handy when you're stuck at a particular weight and the scale hasn't moved for a month.) When nothing else in your life seems to be going right, little victories keep it all in balance and perspective. In so many ways, little victories are Heaven sent.

We've compiled for your consideration a list of little victories experienced not only by us, but also by many others to whom we've spoken. Men, take note, lots of these will apply to you! We included them to cause you to think about what might balance out your fears and doubts about this surgery.

If you go for it, great! If you decide it's not for you, great too! At least you've made the decision and explored your options. If you've already made the decision to go forward with losing weight and getting your life back (by whatever means you choose), here are just a few of the things that will let you know that the journey is a positive one, and that every step is a wonderful new adventure toward an exciting new life:

- Seeing a picture of yourself and not realizing it is actually you!

- Being in pictures at all!!

- Realizing both you and your 5-year-old nephew fit in the recliner as you read him a book.

- Taking a nap on the couch and having room for the cat(s) too.

- Fitting into the stadium seats at sporting events.

- Not being afraid to walk between people in public because you may rub against them.

- Buttoning and zipping up your skirt at the back, not having to do it up in the front and "spin" it to the back.

- Going through the turnstile at the amusement park like everyone else. Not having to be let in through the "gate" on the side.

- Buying jeans that don't have to be purchased in the "work clothing" section of the department store, or the "big and tall men's" shop.

- No longer being referred to as "big guy."

- Knowing your heart isn't going to explode!

- When doing car repairs, being able to lie down on the creeper cart and roll under the car…all the way.

- Strangers actually holding doors for you, or offering to pick up things you have dropped or knocked over.

- Climbing a ladder without fear of it holding you. (Clean those gutters!)

- Not feeling invisible.

- Not wanting to be invisible.

- Strangers acknowledging you with a "hello" who would have never "seen" you before.

- Getting diabetes under control.

- Putting your legs together and feeling the sensation of your knees and ankles touching each other.

- Sitting in the back seat of the car, just because you can.

- Hanging your clothes on regular size hangers and they fit properly.

- Not wearing out your clothes because they "rub" or "pull" at the seams.

- Not wearing out your shoes because you have walked over the sides of them for so long.

- Buying "fun" underwear and pajamas! (Not just the two kinds made in your "other" size.)

- Noticing you actually have a collarbone!

- Getting in the hot tub and not sending a tidal wave of water over the edge.

- The towel fits all the way around!

- Sitting in an airplane seat, crossing your legs, and the tray table STILL lays flat.

- No more racing to the bathroom in complete fear of not making it! (except maybe for dumping syndrome now…)

- Fitting into the ride seats at the amusement park, and the safety bar actually being able to click shut. (Nice to know you won't fall out now when the ride goes upside down…)

- Knowing you can skydive if you want to (but why would you want to?…)

➤ Being set free from the soda pop addiction.

➤ Smaller size hats.

➤ No more back pain!

➤ Being able to dance again.

➤ Fitting in the chair at the hair salon, and not feeling as though the hairstylist is leaning over too far, or contorting himself just to reach your head!

➤ Not secretly "pushing up" with your foot under the chair as your hairstylist or barber pumps the chair to a higher position.

➤ Walking by people who don't recognize you anymore.

➤ Having a waist.

➤ Having a shape that doesn't resemble an appliance!

➤ Finding out you can exercise, and you don't really hate it.

➤ Wearing a smaller size than you did in high school (or junior high!)

➤ Not looking like you dwarf other people in pictures.

➤ The 4-½ hour hamburger, the 6-day pizza, and the 7-week bag of chips.

➤ Taking a shower and not having the shower curtain constantly touching you.

➤ Not feeling self-conscious in the locker room.

➤ Disappearing surgery scars.

➤ Getting off blood pressure medication.

➤ Being able to get down on your knees.

➤ Being able to get up again! By yourself!

➤ Tying your shoes on the top of the shoe, not the side.

➤ Hitting your goal size!

- Hitting your goal weight!

- No longer wrestling yourself into your panty hose.

- Going camping and not being afraid of breaking the aluminum lawn chair you brought to sit in.

- Every new size you fit into.

- The growing space between you and the steering wheel.

- Lower cholesterol.

- Climbing more than two stairs without getting winded, and not using the handrails!

- Taking up less space in bed.

- Taking those flying lessons you always dreamed of because now you fit in the cockpit of the plane.

- Not getting wedged in the bathtub – being able to just sit in the bath tub and get out on your own.

- Running around with your kids in the backyard.

- Feeling worthy again.

- Feeling like a life participant.

- Buying a fishing boat and not being afraid of sinking yourself!

- Sharing the porch swing with your honey, knowing it will hold the two of you, and you both fit with room for the pillows!

- Not having to always use the handicap stall in a public restroom.

- Finding out you don't snore anymore!

- Fitting into an airplane seat and having seatbelt length left over!

- Finding out you wear a smaller shoe size, or you don't need wide shoes anymore.

➤ Feeling proportionate in size to your spouse.

➤ Not feeling like you want to hide when people look at you.

➤ Having people compliment you and not wanting to die.

➤ Feeling you deserve a makeover.

➤ Wearing bright colors.

➤ Joints and bones don't hurt as much.

➤ No more swollen ankles and aching feet.

➤ Being able to get on and ride a motorcycle.

➤ You don't groan in fear at having to pick up dropped items.

➤ No pressure on your bladder.

➤ Not having the arms of a lawn chair (or any other chair) cut into your legs.

➤ Having a BMI that says you're in the "normal" range and you're not "obese" anymore.

➤ Getting a job working with excavating equipment because now you fit in the cab.

➤ Not fearing sliding into a restaurant booth.

➤ Not dripping food on your chest or stomach.

➤ Being able to fit into those little tiny desks or chairs at your kids' school on parent-teacher night!

➤ Going on a date!

➤ Being noticed and appreciated for who you are, not just being noticed for your weight or size.

➤ Actually being able to lean over the sink and brush your teeth.

- Fully realizing that you never have to be fat again because you have control of your weight and your life.

- Standing all the way through a presentation instead of searching frantically for a place to sit down.

- Fitting all the way under an umbrella.

- Riding a snowmobile and wearing an actual snowmobile suit!

- Not shopping at the end of the rack (and knowing there's no place else to go...)

- Finding new stores you can shop in.

- Realizing you can actually see your ears when you look at yourself in the mirror.

- Not feeling like you have to make fun of yourself to fit in, or to make the joke about yourself before others do.

- Learning not to celebrate everything with food, and getting other people in your life to accept that as well.

- Climbing the ladder to your son or daughter's tree house.

- Not being exhausted all the time.

- Going ice fishing with your friends and not being afraid of breaking through the ice and drowning the lot of you!

- Being able to physically pick up your kids.

- Having your kids be able to sit on your lap.

- Having a lap!

- Fitting in the seat of your beloved riding lawn tractor, and not have the steering wheel cut into your stomach.

- Discovering you have hip bones.

- Hugging someone and actually feeling the hug.

- No longer wedging yourself into the "porta-john" on the work site.

- No more insensitive comments or remarks about your weight or your size.

- No fat prejudice at interviews or on dates.

- Feeling like a normal size person and accepting what's normal for you.

- Flirting!!

- Being able to itch places you could never reach before.

- Waistbands and bra straps not cutting in anymore.

- Being able to take a really deep breath.

- Getting hit on at the bookstore!!

- Climbing up into your 4X4 heavy-duty pickup truck and not needing extra handles and home-built step blocks to get in.

- Passing the junk food aisle in the grocery store and feeling okay about it.

- Knowing you have kicked the fast food habit.

- No cravings/compulsions/obsessions for food.

- Fitting into goal clothing.

- A whole new sex life.

- Feeling good about wearing jewelry.

- Being able to pull into small parking spaces because you don't need to get the car door open as far.

- Being able to buy a scale.

- Not being afraid to get on the scale!

- Riding a bike and not having the seat go up your butt!!

- Fitting into theater and auditorium seating.

- Being able to buy tickets for the "cheap seats" because you know you can make the hike up there.

- Being able to sit in the middle seat on an airplane (but still…why would you want to!)

- Getting your dimples back or discovering you have them.

- Not feeling like you have to apologize for yourself.

- Discovering your fingers have gotten longer and thinner.

- Playing sports again, not just watching it.

- Actually wanting to look in a mirror.

- Being able to get up off low, cushy furniture.

- Breathing properly all through the night (getting rid of sleep apnea).

- Getting down on the floor with your children to play with the slot car track.

- Not feeling self-conscious when walking away from people because they might be getting a rear view.

- Tucking your shirt into your jeans, and feeling good about how you look.

- No longer feeling like you have to wear a jacket because you're self-conscious about your big rear end.

- Taking that cross-country cycling tour.

- Going to the doctor's office and knowing you won't have to deal with any more Fat Nazi doctors!

- Not being agoraphobic anymore.

- Getting on the elevator and not looking at the weight restriction sign.

- Being able to share the armrest with the person next to you.

- Looking down and seeing the shadow of a normal sized person.

➤ Riding in go-carts!

➤ Not having to look for the closest parking space anymore, because you can easily walk the distance from the car to the store.

➤ Being at a size that it becomes noticeable to people when you've only lost 10 pounds.

➤ Having your honey (or anyone else) be able to get his or her arms more than all the way around you.

Chapter Nine

⟵ S E P A R A T I O N   A N X I E T Y ⟶

Julie M. Janeway

Karen J. Sparks

As the title might suggest, this chapter will address some of the things you'll be leaving behind along your journey. When Karen and I started this process, we both thought we'd be quite happy to leave behind just about everything (husband, cats, family, and friends not included), in order to craft new lives for ourselves as thin people. What we found was that saying good-bye isn't as easy as one might think — not even saying good-bye to the pounds.

In the beginning, every pound that disappears is like a little gift from Heaven. After all, you have so many more to lose, and isn't that the purpose of all this? At this point you're concentrating on watching the numbers finally go down on the scale (not up anymore!), and on recovering from surgery.

As the pounds come off though, you'll go through periods of shrinkage that are very extreme. Literally you can shrink a size over a weekend. You will have worn a piece of clothing on Monday, then the following Monday, it will be radically too big. It's a very strange phenomenon, and more than a little frustrating. But, more on that later. We call these (appropriately) "shrinks."

But there comes a time when you go through a shrink, and this time you notice some major difference in yourself. Some drastic change appears, like you can see your ears again when you look at yourself head on in the mirror, or maybe you've shrunk into a piece of goal clothing, or you notice that your hands don't even look like your hands anymore. Maybe it's that your feet have shrunk and you can't keep your shoes on anymore. These realizations are mile-markers along the journey.

So, with each little realization (and there will be many), you're hit squarely in the face with the fact that you're getting thinner, and the fact that you used to be really big (or really, really big as the case may be). All of a sudden you find yourself in an introspective mood, re-examining why and how you got to where you started, where you are now, and where you're going.

This introspection examines each pound you carried around for so long. Each pound came as a result of some rejection, some hurtful remark, or some blow to your self-esteem. In fact, they became part of the insulation that kept you separated from the prickly nature of the world. Many of us wore our weight like a sandwich board that said, "Stay away from me. You can't hurt me anymore."

Of course we also knew, that the louder and more obvious we made that statement, the more the world felt entitled to comment and editorialize — and the more it hurt. It's a vicious cycle. What's a person to do? (And another pizza would bite the dust....)

You begin to re-examine each stage of your life and your weight gain. You examine the pain that accompanied those pounds, and you meet it head on as the pounds drop away. It's not so much the pounds that are hard to lose, but the pieces of the life they represent that really hits you.

Dealing with each pound and its attendant emotional injuries as they come off, you begin the emotional ride of a lifetime. As you shrink into your clothes from days gone past, it brings up a whole new era of painful memories with which to deal. Each compliment about how much "better you look now," seems to be a bittersweet mix of compliment and criticism. The new little victories of everyday life still sit in stark contrast to the memories of failure, rejection, disapproval, self-deprecation, self-doubt, and denial.

But, it's not all bad. Every day there's still elation with another pound gone, and the knowledge that you have dealt with its emotional struggle. Those pounds and those struggles won't control you anymore. The memories will always be there, but with each day comes a strengthened resolve not to succumb to those emotional forces, and an increasing sense of empowerment never to let those weight-related emotional injuries happen to you again.

You'll bring the unaddressed pain out of the basement. You'll examine it, try it on, confront its ill-fit, fold it, put it in a box, label it, and tuck it nicely into the attic of your psyche. Some memories and scars are faster and easier to deal with than others, but that's pretty much the process that transpires with each couple of pounds lost.

With each pound lost, and each new change in size comes an exploration and re-examination of self-perception and self-concept. "Self-perception" is how you see yourself, physically, mentally, and socially. "Self-concept" includes self-perception, but also includes your idea of who you are as person, what you bring to this planet and this existence.

You will struggle with self-perception. It will change many times through the course of this journey. You may have thought of yourself as heavy, but smart. Maybe heavy, but clever. How about heavy, but fun? Maybe creative, or attractive (if not beautiful or handsome), kind, thoughtful, loving, shy, or caring. But always fat, heavy, or overweight. For many people, their self-perception degrades, and they simply think of themselves as "fat, dumb, ugly, stupid, and unacceptable," or some version thereof. This is the problem with self-perception, when one characteristic tends to dictate all others.

As you begin to take away the concepts of "fat," "heavy," and "overweight," you must re-evaluate whether or not you are still "shy," "quiet," or "reserved." Are you still fun? Are you still introverted? Are you really dumb? Are you beautiful or handsome now? This will continue to change and morph as you lose more and more weight. Your self-perception will continue to change along with your entire self-concept.

The famed sociologist Charles Horton Cooley (another Michigander…) said that the concept of "self" is developed from our interaction with others. He coined the term the "looking-glass self," and summarized the concept with this couplet: "Each to each a looking-glass, Reflects the other that doth pass."[1]

The looking-glass self contains three elements: 1) we imagine how we appear to those around us; 2) we interpret others' reactions; and, 3) we develop a self-concept.[2]

As people insecure about our weight we imagine how we appear to others. We may perceive that if someone is staring at us, it *has* to be because we are fat, not because we are striking, or humorous, or just standing in front of the sign they are trying to read.

As people unhappy because of our weight, we interpret others' reactions or lack of reactions. We may perceive that because no one is looking at us, that it must be a negative thing as well. Our interpretation of thin people getting asked out on dates more often than fat people (or so we surmise) is that we are not acceptable as dating partners, and therefore *everything* about us must be unacceptable.

We interpret many reactions correctly and many incorrectly. And, it's important to note, self-concepts don't have to be based on accurate evaluations, perceptions, or interpretations of what others' may think of us, and how they may react. In fact, more times than not, they are incorrect, and based on our own self-doubts and insecurities – like being overweight.

Whether they were right or wrong, we may have taken the collection of all those interpretations and perceptions of what we thought people were thinking and trying to tell us, and strung them together like beads on a necklace. Our necklaces were then wrapped around our throats and became our self-concepts. For many of us, our negative and inaccurate self-concepts veritably choked us to death. On this journey, that will quickly change.

Your physical change will be drastic, and your self-concept will change drastically as well. If you've always been a stay-at-home parent, partially because of weight, but mostly because of self-concept, then losing the weight will cause you to reassess whether you might want to go out now and get a job. Maybe you will, maybe you won't.

Maybe you'll find that being a stay-at-home parent is okay, but perhaps you'll be inspired to join some parent-teacher groups because you have so many ideas for improving your kids' school, and you have the newfound confidence to promote them.

Similarly, for those who've never ventured far into the dating world because of a series of hurtful reactions and events, many of you have resigned yourselves to the fact that you were just meant to be alone. You've developed a concept of yourself as a single person, and a person for whom intimate personal relationships just aren't in the cards. Well, when you lose the weight, many of those barriers will be gone. You may find yourself in a bookstore or grocery store one day, and someone will be staring or smiling at you, and subtly trying to get your attention. And NO, I'm not talking about the salesperson motioning to get you to move to checkout number five!

You may find that people want to get to know you, or maybe even ask you on a date. Accept if you want to — unless you're married. The challenge for you is to leave the hurt behind. Don't let it control you anymore. Don't drag into your new self-concept the resentment toward those who previously rejected you because of your weight. Don't let it hamper your new life. Learn to live in the moment, and put all the rest behind you. Learn to think of yourself as a renewed and vibrant person worth getting to know, and worthy of being loved. Learn to deal with yourself that way as well.

Learning to value and respect yourself is what we term "self-esteem." You will see almost daily improvements in your self-esteem, but beware the "fat day." Just because you're losing weight and feeling better, doesn't mean that every time you look in the mirror you're going to love what you see. There will be days that you'll see someone you like much better than the person you saw the day before, and on other days (when you're tired, or stressed, or a little under the weather), you may see someone who's still fat, or lumpy, or misshapen.

Beware of those days. Let the day happen, but don't let it affect your new self-esteem. Tell yourself, "I will feel differently tomorrow." And most likely, you will. (But, if you feel down and depressed for more than a week, you need to call your doctor's office as your high protein, lower carb diet may have caused your serotonin levels to drop too far, and some mild anti-depressants may be required for a short time.)

So, you're going to deal with the excitement of new and improved self-esteem, self-perception, and self-concept — all of which we may collectively refer to as your sense of "self" or sense of "identity." And it can be a really fun ride. But there are some things about which you should be aware.

At some point your sense of "identity" and "self-concept" may begin to run head on into someone else's idea of your "identity," or who they think you're supposed to be. This has happened to more people than I care to think about.

I talked to one young woman who told me of her two life-long friends. They'd been friends since kindergarten, and they were coincidentally (or not so coincidentally), all overweight. This young woman decided to have weight loss surgery, much to the consternation and dismay of her two friends. Despite the fact that she was one of those surgery mill cases I talked about in the first chapter, she still managed to lose the weight.

As she shrunk through her second size in about six weeks, one of her two friends completely stopped speaking to her. When asked why, the friend stated that the young woman losing the weight thought she was better than the other two now. When asked how she came to this conclusion, the angry friend said it was obvious because the young woman who had surgery wouldn't go out to eat with them anymore, and she was just a "little too happy" about wearing a smaller size than they did. And so, a friendship was lost because one person could not accept or keep up with the other person's rapidly changing lifestyle, self-esteem, and self-concept.

It's happened to Karen and me as well: family members who don't know how to deal with you because you've changed; co-workers who are finding that they can't dump all the overtime work on you anymore because you actually have a life to attend to now; and, friends who can't deal with the fact that you're not at their beck and call to solve all their problems for them. It's a whole new deal. There's actually a name for this: it's called "role exit," and it comes from a sociological theory developed by a man named Erving Goffman.

Erving Goffman created a theory he called "dramaturgy," to explain interactions between human beings. All the dramaturgy theory says is that life is like a play. We're either on stage (out there interacting with people), or we're off stage (doing things in private).[3]

If we're on stage, we've adopted roles like student, wife, lawyer, sister, father, Aunt, friend, teacher, boss, store clerk, or whatever. With these roles come props to use, and a costume or series of costumes to wear. In other words we dress the part in addition to acting the part. What also comes with our roles is a determined way of interacting with other people in their roles.

If you've seen a play or movie ten times, you always expect the characters to dress the same way, say the same lines, and interact the same way. You're very uncomfortable when you see a remake of the play or movie, and it's radically different. (Ask Leonardo DiCaprio about "Romeo and Juliet"....)

Imagine a remake of "Casablanca" with Chris Rock in Humphrey Bogart's role, or "The Phantom of the Opera" starring Jackie Chan as a martial arts blazing Phantom, or even Kathy Bates starring as Rizzo in a reprisal of "Grease." Get it? Not that it can't or shouldn't be done, but it is really outside of what you expect, and what is comfortable for you. Because it's not comfortable, you'll naturally resist, or even become angry, and want things to be the way "they should be!"

So it is with real life. We adopt for ourselves particular roles – Rock of Gibraltar for everyone, white knight and rescuer, fixer of all things, single person, confessor and confidante, home-body, the one who's always prepared and can/will handle everything, frumpy introvert, or maybe even "doormat." Others adopt their roles accordingly, and they expect that if their roles don't change, neither should ours. We should continue to interact as we always have. They just don't understand why we can't get with the program!!

But that's not what happens. As your self-perception and self-concept change, so do your limitations, fears, and doubts. One by one, the roles you've chosen for yourself based on your weight, limitations, fears, and doubts, begin to fall away. New roles are adopted in their place because interaction with the world changes and increases, and that puts you "on stage" more than you were before.

Our new roles involve taking care of ourselves a little more. Our new roles involve doing the things we couldn't before. Our new roles often involve making up for lost time, if possible. What they don't involve is loving the people in our lives any less. They don't involve a change in our basic values, beliefs, and personal ethics. They don't involve a change in our core being.

But often others can't see that, and conflict arises. This conflict arises from "role exit." You're leaving a particular role either to play a different role in the same play, or a different role in a whole new play. You may take on a whole new role within your family, for example, as leader and visionary instead of follower and workhorse. That's taking on a new role, but staying in the same play.

Quitting your job because you realize you don't deserve, and no longer have to accept the abuse that is heaped on you day after day, is an example of adopting a new role and moving to a new play. Both are hard, and be prepared for the conflict. Oh, the crying, wailing, and gnashing of teeth that will go on!!

Taking on a new role and staying in the same play (or drama, as the case may be), is especially hard if that play happens to be your family. Your role in the family has been determined over a lot of years. Your role may be as the" fixer of all things." That may be your role because when you were heavy you didn't have much of a life, and you were always expected to be around to fix everyone's problems. Maybe that expectation didn't come from others, but instead you wanted to be the fixer because in your mind it gave people something to love about you, and a reason to be wanted and needed.

Maybe you were the "Ann Landers" of the family, as my mother would say. You might be expected to be everyone's therapist, and we all know therapists aren't supposed to bring their own problems to the proverbial couch. Whatever the role, you may find yourself changing it in favor of roles you've always wanted to play, and that's okay, no matter how others may whine about it.

This process is all about dealing with your own stuff. And, as we've said many times in this book, this is a journey that is wholly selfish, and just for you. So, it necessitates you leaving (even temporarily) roles like this, and boy others may not be happy about it!! The trick is to keep reassuring them that you don't love them any less, and that you aren't becoming a whole new person on the inside, just the outside. (You're just changing a little on the inside; tidying things up a bit, if you will.) You need to assure them that you just want to experience life a little more, and they're more than welcome to join you.

Let them know that this is hard for you too, as you're very accustomed to the roles you've played. Also, let them know that part of the reason you adopted the roles in the first place was because of those limitations, fears, and doubts associated with your weight. Maybe they'll understand that the weight is really the driving force here.

Discuss with them how much weight has affected every facet of your life. Let them know that it is still going to affect every facet of your life until you're finally comfortable with yourself. Then you'll decide what roles you want to play in the long term, and things will settle down a bit. Let them know that the flux and frustration is not permanent.

And flux and frustration there will be. Not only are you going through separation anxiety from the old you to the new you, but you will go through other forms of separation anxiety as well; forms such as separating from celebrating all events with food. That's a hard one because our culture, and in fact so many of the world's cultures celebrate with food.

It's not that you can't ever be in the room with a birthday cake again, or you have to skip Christmas dinner. What you do need to change is celebrating your favorite sports team's regular season win against the last ranked team, by going out for pizza and beer. Similarly, the 80% off shoe sale at the mall is not cause for cookies at Mrs. Fields®!

Although you'll be able to make this change fairly easily (because you'll experience dumping as a result of these indulgences), others in your life may have a harder time. They need to understand that you're not imposing on them any sort of penalty for your new lifestyle. They're welcome to continue celebrating whatever they need to, in the manner to which they've become accustomed, and you'll be happy to participate — just not in eating inappropriate food. Sounds easy, doesn't it? Yeah, well... wait until you try this for the first time....

You may find family members or others who are very insulted that you chose not to eat a piece of birthday cake or a particular dish they made. Or you may find that people want to change all the holiday dishes to make sure you can eat them. Although that's nice and very well meaning, it's not necessary.

Tell them not to change the traditional holiday meal (or any meal) to accommodate you. You'll pick around, and find what you can and can't eat. Everything should remain the same for everyone else's sake, as well as yours. Tell them, "Just don't bug me to eat more, or harass me about what I am eating, or how long it takes to eat it." We hope for your sake, they'll understand. Some will, some won't.

I'M NOT DONE YET !

Remember the story we told you previously of the young woman and her two life-long friends? After her surgery she still hung out with them, and did everything she used to do. She just wouldn't be their eating partner anymore. She went with them to restaurants at first, but she found it boring and annoying to sit there while they ate food she knew she (and they), shouldn't be eating.

She finally stopped going out to the restaurants, but she still wanted to continue hanging out and doing other things together. The one friend simply could not accept that. It was the friend's problem entirely, but instead of dealing with it, she dumped it back on the young woman who was trying to change her life and eating habits. Not cool. But that's the kind of stuff that happens. You just have to realize whose problem it really is, and don't take responsibility for other people's issues. You'll have enough issues to deal with on your own. Trust us on that.

Similarly, here's something that is a constant battle in my house. My husband, Matt, is 6'3" tall, about 190 pounds, and he's built like a swimmer. The man has the metabolism of a hummingbird, and he has to eat like an elephant to keep weight on, let alone increase his weight. (Man, that always just ticked me right off…) Karen calls him the "ten-toed stomach."

Matt is a very hard worker, and one of those people who can never sit down. He's always working at something, so when he wants to eat, he wants to EAT! He, like most other men, is on the see-food diet. He sees it, he eats it. And usually, he'll eat all, or the better part of all of it. The man can eat an entire package of Oreos® in one sitting if he has enough milk to dip them in, and a good movie to watch!

The problem arises when Matt decides to eat everything that is readily available or microwaveable (the man simply WILL NOT cook), and then he absent-mindedly starts in on the few things that I know I can eat successfully. It is at this point that the battle lines are drawn.

Because I can't eat very much in one sitting, things will either go in the refrigerator for another meal, or go back in the cupboard as the case may be; at least that's the theory. When I make dinner, I'll serve my portion, and then Matt will come in later and get his. The issue is that when I have cooked what I think is enough for at least two more meals after the night's dinner, Matt simply thinks the rest *is* his dinner! One night I cooked six pork chops. I ate one, and thought there'd be at least two left over for me to eat as other meals. Matt thought otherwise. He ate all five pork chops. (Sigh!... they don't call them Man-imals for nothing….)

Now I can hear what you're saying: "Serve yours and his at the same time, and then he'll know how much he can eat." Duh!!! I tried that! It didn't work. He just went back and got more until it was gone! So you say, "Then serve the plates, and put the rest away before you hand him his." Duh, again!!! He went to the fridge, got it out, and threw the rest in the microwave. If I could figure out how to cook exactly the right amount, and not leave one of the two of us hungry, I'd be golden. I have scientists at MIT working on it….

Maybe he always ate like that. Maybe I just never noticed until now because my food portions are so much smaller. I don't know. If I buy bananas, I can only eat one every couple of days. I might get one out of the whole bunch because Matt decides that over the course of one day, he needs to eat three. I can't keep up with that, nor can I go banana, or grocery shopping every two days!

All I know is that I now have to stash food like a pack rat around the house so I can be assured of getting just *some* of the food I know I can eat (apples behind my computer, granola bars in my underwear drawer, bananas in my briefcase. I haven't quite figured out where to stash cooked chicken breasts though, so they remain vulnerable to Matt-attack in the refrigerator).

I've explained to him that I just can't keep up with that level of food intake, and that I have to know that certain types of foods are there when I need them. He understands, but then he gets very upset when I catch him absentmindedly delving into my box of low-fat crackers, and ask him to stop eating my food! I can't win for losing here. I can't even imagine what it would be like if I had Matt and children on top of it! I'd starve to death….

So you see, there's a form of separation anxiety that occurs with the food in your house as well. You used to take for granted that you'd get your share, or at least it would be there when you wanted it. Say good-bye to getting your share. Heck, for a long time you won't even be sure what your share should be!

Like I said, I don't know whether he always ate like that, or I'm just noticing now because my food portions are smaller. Maybe it's because food controls me now more than it ever did. Food and its purpose in keeping me alive and healthy are always at the forefront of my thoughts. I'm not a person who likes to cook or bake (a genetic anomaly according to my sister and father), and in a way I'm glad, because if I were a person whose life and enjoyment centered around making elaborate food, I don't know how I'd cope.

Although Karen doesn't necessarily make elaborate food, she can if she wants to. She really enjoys cooking, baking, and even candy making, and she's incredibly good at it. She reported that she found it strange, and a little difficult this past Christmas when she and her nephew went on their traditional all-day cookie baking and candy-making binge.

Now, you have to understand, we're talking Mrs. Claus, North Pole level set-up here — thirty to forty dozen cookies in six varieties, ten pounds of peanut brittle, chocolates, and a host of other (killer) goodies. Previously, she'd always enjoyed snacking on her own handiwork as she made it. This year she simply made it. She and her nephew still had fun, but only he got to lick the spoons. What she normally would have kept for herself, she boxed up and gave to friends. (The rest appears on Christmas Day at their big family get-together, as a gift from the elves. Isn't that cute? The kids love it. They're such a Norman Rockwell family.)

She didn't really say that the experience wasn't fun, but I think some of the fun came from eating all the good things she'd made. Certainly, her memories were now different from the actual experience, and she had to think about whether or not that was a good or bad thing. That phenomenon is called "cognitive dissonance," in case you care.[4] These are the types of separations from your previous life that you begin to notice, and some cause more anxiety than others.

I'll tell you what else you may notice (and for a while you may have a hard time with it for some reason): how much other people eat, and wondering where they put it. I never saw this one coming, because frankly I was always so involved in my own eating, I never stopped long enough to notice other people. Now I do, and it's a little disconcerting.

One day, my husband was starving (what else is new?), and he wanted to stop off at his favorite all-you-can-eat buffet restaurant (translation: grazing station). We went in, and I didn't bother ordering anything, because after this surgery there is no possible way you can get your $11.99 worth of food out of the place. You'd have to stay for a week, and pack food in a suitcase to go. (This goes for Mother's Day buffets, Easter Sunday buffets, Thanksgiving, cruises, and any other event or situation that includes gargantuan amounts of available food.)

I sat there while he stuffed his lean frame full of food, and strangely it didn't bother me that I wasn't eating with him. But what did bother me was watching all the other people. They had unbelievably enormous amounts of food in front of them. I watched them go back for three, four, five trips to the buffet.

I couldn't believe how much they put in their mouths at one time. Each forkful was about half of what my entire meal would be now! Did I used to do that? Sadly, yes. How is it that I didn't just explode? How is it that they don't just explode? It's the weirdest thing, and it still bothers me.

I would never in a million years say anything to anyone, but I can't help watching people eat every time I'm out. It fascinates me. Karen too. And everyone else we've talked to as well. We're all enthralled with America's eating.

It's hard to deal with the fact that you used to eat this way; that you would stuff as much salad in your mouth in one forkful, as you now eat in total with your entire meal. That's very hard to get your head around. Some days you'll be very grateful that's not you anymore, and on other days it will just be depressing. It's hard to separate yourself from all that, and stop mulling it over every time you watch people eat — or every time you eat.

Case in point: If you're wondering how we came to determine that the all-you-can-eat buffet is no longer a cost-efficient, or practical night out, well, let us tell you about our little experience with that.

Karen and I were at yet another conference, this time in Ann Arbor. We'd broken out of the conference, and hit the ground running at all the local discount stores. At one point, later in the afternoon, we determined that we simply had to stop to eat. Protein rules your life. So, we decided that the best thing to do was to go somewhere that the food was already made so we could save time and get back to big-game bargain hunting, and "important woman-business." Fast food is generally out unless it's a true emergency because the choices are limited, and you have to do too much dismantling. Then we spied "the buffet."

Fond thoughts of being able to eat yourself into a stupor at "the buffet" came flooding back to both of us. All reason was temporarily suspended. We pulled in, quickly paid our $11.99 each, and headed for the steam tables. So many kinds of protein to choose from! And other goodies too like vegetables, and salad, and potatoes. We didn't even give a thought to the desserts or the fried stuff, so I guess not ALL rational thought had flown out the window, but certainly our eyes were bigger than our teeny weeny little stomachs. Our emotional eating memories were taking over.

We each grabbed some baked chicken, and roast beef, and ham, and whatever else looked like it had protein in it. We grabbed some iced tea, veritably raced for the table, and dug in. Now, let's just stop right there. There is just so much wrong with this picture, I don't even know where to start. What were we thinking???

First, we'd taken too much food. Second, it was all covered in gravy or sauce. Third, we were mesmerized by the food, and were eating on memory. Fourth, we were eating too fast. Fifth, we weren't chewing enough. Sixth, we were drinking while eating. And seventh, we'd paid $11.99 each, and we still thought we could get our money's worth. FOOLS!!!

We both ploughed through the first ten bites or so of our respective plates, and then it hit. Auto Eject!! We both made ourselves so sick, we actually laid down on the seats in the booth. (The good news being we'd lost enough weight to be able to lay down on the seats of the booth!)

Oh, and it was a bad one too. I don't know which one of us was greener, but Kermit had nothing on either of us! Fortune had smiled, however, in that we had serendipitously chosen a table near the bathroom. Thank God, for small favors. (Unfortunately, they don't keep pillows tucked behind their toilets for people like us.)

It took about an hour and a half before either one of us returned to some normal skin color. I know people were very afraid. You could tell by the odd looks, and the hushed tones that accompanied long sideways stares. I'm sure we weren't exactly a raving endorsement for the restaurant either. I'm surprised they didn't throw us out.

We sat there, and sat there, and sat there. We kept telling each other that we had to eat more because we hadn't yet consumed enough protein (like either one of us cared at that point!). So, we picked a little here, and picked a little there. By that time the food was cold, so we ditched it and got some new stuff that was warm, and not as drowned in gravy or sauce. Amazingly enough, neither of us felt guilty about wasting the food. After all we'd spent $11.99 each, and it was quickly becoming apparent that we weren't going to be able to eat even $2.99 worth of food in total.

We continued to pick a bit here and there. What we found ourselves doing in the meantime, was watching all the other people in the restaurant. They were more than getting their money's worth. Again, we couldn't understand where they were putting it all. Then we'd look at each other and remember when we used to do the same thing, or worse.

Amid watching others consume $35.00 worth of food, and dealing with the fact that we were subsidizing at least six people's dinners, we simply became consumed with how much money we'd wasted. We were determined to remember this experience, and we were determined to get at least most of our money's worth, one way or another.

All in all, we sat there for four and a half hours. We managed to get out of there with two dozen cookies hidden in purses, coat pockets, and one of our calendar portfolios, that we proudly brought home and presented to Matt. We figured that about made the restaurant and us even.

This experience caused us both to examine the fact that we kind of had to separate ourselves from places and events that involved large quantities of food, or inappropriate foods. Drive-thrus, buffets, and sometimes even regular restaurant meals are generally just not worth it.

Fast food drive-thrus are rarely an acceptable choice anymore because even if you order a plain chicken breast, it might still cost you $4.00! Salads are okay, but the dressings generally aren't, and pretty much nothing else is acceptable. Buffets? Well, we've discussed that. Regular meals at restaurants *always* involve bringing at least half home, and then it just dies a cold, lonely death in the fridge before it goes in the garbage. We both had to figure out how to separate from these memories, patterns, and choices, while still living a fairly normal life, and interacting with the world on a social basis.

Making these types of separations is like trying to adapt your personal subculture to living within the dominant culture. You have to live with the big structure of things: restaurants, and food-laden events never go away. But you also have to be true to what you need to do: eat smaller portions, waste less money, and not eat inappropriate food. Separating from one's culture, even a little, is a difficult thing. Ask anyone who's moved halfway around the world.

And speaking of separating from things…(or being separated as the case may be…), we now come to the issue of the anxiety associated with giving up material things. By material things we mean, clothes, shoes, and accessories. Now, if you're a man reading this, I would not stop at this point if I were you. We realize that men don't generally have the emotional attachment to their clothing that women do (or, do they…?), but this will apply in part to you as well. You *will* experience some of this stuff. Trust us.

The last thing in the world I expected to be an issue for me, was shrinking out of my clothes. I know Karen echoes these thoughts, because she's sitting here, reading over my shoulder, nodding her head. If you'd asked either one of us what we were most looking forward to, one of the top five answers was wearing a smaller size, and getting rid of my "fat clothes." Oh, how we were both looking forward to that!

Well, we're here to testify that it can be every bit as glorious an experience as you've ever imagined it to be, and more. The celebrations we've had! The happy dances we've done in stores! The hooting and hollering that has gone on in dressing rooms! My, my, my, what fools we've made of ourselves! But here's the ugly side of it.

Because weight loss surgery causes you to lose a large amount of weight very quickly, more quickly than you've ever experienced, you cannot prepare for the pace at which you will shrink. You will have "shrinks" at the strangest times (for women most likely right after your monthly cycle, but any other time your body feels like it too), and you won't necessarily shrink evenly.

You may find that one day your clothes fit fine, and two days later you put on the same clothes and the top or bottom is now too big. Think about it. You're losing between 15 and 30 pounds a month for the first six months or so. That's a lot of weight to drop, and what remains then has to shift around, and get resituated.

Additionally, with fat it's kind of a last on, first off sort of thing. Wherever you put the weight on last is generally where it will come off first. So for Karen and me, we shrank more and faster on the top than on the bottom (typical for many women), and when you are shrinking unevenly in the top and bottom, it's hard to keep up, and hard to know what size you really are.

So the moral of the story here is, "shrinks," although appreciated and the purpose of the entire process, are unpredictable, and they can cause some pretty serious clothing crises. Let me give you a few examples

I had several sizes of clothes to shrink into. Problem: I hit each particular size during a time of year for which I had no appropriate clothing. Let me explain. I shrank into a size 24, but the last time I was a size 24, it was Winter, so the majority of my clothes were Winter clothes. When I shrunk into size 24, it was unfortunately, Spring. I shrunk past an entire wardrobe of clothes I never got to wear. So, I had to go out and find clothes that fit me. $Cha-ching!$

I bought some clothes, and when I shrunk into a size 22, I had a few Spring and Summer pieces I could wear, thank goodness. What I didn't have was a pair of navy pants. Navy pants were particularly difficult to find during the summer of 2004 (why???), and it wasn't until about July that I finally found a pair (now in size 20), and a bargain at only $14.00 too!

I bought them on a Sunday (that's important to the story). They were cropped pants so that meant I couldn't wear them to work, but I was looking forward to wearing them the following weekend. The following Saturday I put the pants on and let out one horrific scream. My husband came running. "What's wrong? What's the matter?" he stammered. I was so hopping mad, I couldn't even get words out. Finally, I hissed, "These stupid pants are too big!" I'd shrunk during the week, and the pants were now almost three inches too big in the waist. I was so ticked off!

My husband was trying to be supportive, and of course he missed the point entirely. He said, "Well, isn't that what you wanted? To lose the weight?" Well, duh!!

But, I hunted all Spring and Summer for these pants! They were a phenomenal bargain! I love them! I never even got to wear them, and now they have to go back to the store!! Don't you get it???? Of course, he didn't.

That scene has repeated so many times at my house, I've lost count. It happened virtually the same way one day with a belt. The belt fit a week before, and that day, because I was in a hurry, the belt was now two and a half inches past the last hole. I went screaming into the living room, bellowing for Matt. He came in dazed and bewildered at my freak-out over a belt. Again, he simply thought I should be thrilled I'd shrunk again. He plainly didn't realize that once again, it was at an inconvenient time.

Now don't get me wrong. I was grateful for each of those shrinks, and I celebrated those losses appropriately. But, I'm telling you, they do come at the most annoying times sometimes. So, that's one type of separation anxiety over clothes, and here's another: separating from clothes with emotional attachments.

I started weeding my closet about every two weeks once I started losing the weight. I figured, once I'm out of it, I'm out of it for good. There's no going back, baby. Of course, I kept a few things to go to the tailor to be resized. If you don't you'll simply end up naked. But then there were things to which I had an emotional attachment, and I didn't want to let them go. One of those things was the long velvet jacket my mother bought me for Christmas, 2001.

I'd barely been out of the hospital after my accident, and my mom bought me this beautiful velvet jacket with rhinestone buttons as a Christmas present. I so loved it, and I know it cost her more money than she really had to spend. More importantly, I felt thin in it. (I *wasn't* thin in it, but I felt thin!)

But those weren't the only reasons I didn't want to get rid of it. The biggest reason was because that was what I was wearing on New Year's Eve, when Matt asked me to marry him. I took it and had it cut down twice, but then it simply got to a point that it couldn't be cut down anymore. It's a size 20 now, and I'm a 14. I'll never be able to wear it again. Yet, I still can't let it go.

Similarly, and maybe worse, I can't even bring myself to look at my wedding dress. I was a size 28 by the time I got married, and although I designed my dress, and it was beautiful, it wasn't really the dress of my dreams because I wasn't the size I wanted to be. Now, I'm actually the size I always wanted to be when I got married. I simply can't bring myself to take the dress out and look at it, let alone try it on. I just know I won't be able to control the tears.

It doesn't have to be clothing that has life changing memories attached though, it can just be things you've really enjoyed. Karen and I both have many pieces that we just loved that have gone by the wayside. They were mainly pieces we'd hunted so very hard to find (being in plus –sizes and all), and we actually liked them, felt good in them, and felt just a little bit like normal people in them. It's hard to say good-bye to something that made you feel good, even just for a short while.

It's hard to say good-bye to your favorite shoes when your feet shrink. It's hard to say good-bye to clothes that seem too long now, because you've shrunk enough that the proportions of plus-size clothes are just all wrong. It's hard to say good-bye to your favorite jeans because they're all "broken in" in just the right places. It's hard to say good-bye to jewelry that appears enormous now, when it was such a treasured find, and important piece of your wardrobe before.

And the sad part is that you don't just say good-bye once. You keep doing it over and over again as you shrink through the sizes. You may shrink into a pair of jeans you've had for ten years. Getting those goal jeans on is what you've been waiting for. They finally fit, and life is just grand. Then three weeks later, they're too big, and you only got to wear them twice. Say good-bye again.

Maybe you've bought yourself something new, maybe even something you've always wanted. Wear it quickly, because you'll have to say good-bye soon enough. This is very hard stuff!!! Especially, when you never get to wear something! Karen and I have just too many things that still have the tags attached; thus the garage sale mentioned in Chapter Two.

Each of us has things we value and cherish, whether it be a wedding dress, a beloved college t-shirt, or a tattered and torn pair of comfy sneakers. Each of you will go through the separation anxiety that comes with saying good-bye to your favorite articles of clothing, shoes, and accessories. You may not think you have any attachments, but mark our words: you do.

When you make changes in your life as extreme as the ones that result from weight loss surgery, you begin to examine all the things in life to which you are attached. We've told you before that this process involves learning new skills, one of which is living a different lifestyle. But another is learning new coping strategies, and facing emotional issues with strength and courage. We hope that letting you in on some of the situations we've encountered will provide you with a little more strength and courage to face your own.

I am not going to limit myself
just because people won't accept the fact
that I can do something else.

DOLLY PARTON

Dr. Randal S. Baker and his family

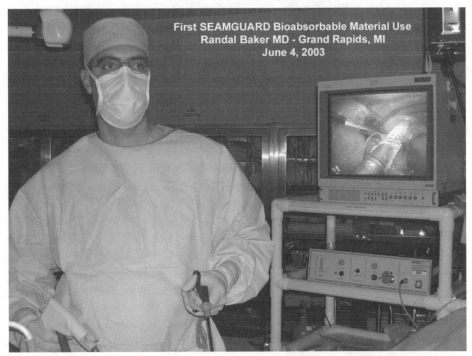

First SEAMGUARD Bioabsorbable Material Use
Randal Baker MD - Grand Rapids, MI
June 4, 2003

Dr. Baker using the Seamguard® product for the first time anywhere on the planet!

Julie's "before" pictures

Julie's "after" pictures

Karen's "before & after" pictures

Karen's family

Julie's fur-child, Smuggy

Julie's fur-child, Smudgie

Judith Brown Clarke

Scott H. Glass, M.S., M.A., L.L.P.

Carrie A. Liebrock, R.D. and Willow

Chapter Ten

NO GIRLS ALLOWED!

Randal S. Baker M.D., F.A.C.S.
Julie M. Janeway
Karen J. Sparks

More and more men are having this surgery these days, and we thought it was about time to bring the issues that men deal with out into the light. The vast majority of information lurking around out there deals with women who are choosing to have the surgery, and so this chapter is dedicated to the guys and the difficulties they encounter by virtue of the fact they were born male (and no, that is not a character flaw). This is not a new millennium version of the "he-man woman-haters club," but let's just say you have to have a "Y" chromosome to join.

We interviewed a number of male weight loss surgery patients, both from my practice and from other medical institutions as well. Some recently had their surgery, and some were as far as two years out. Some were young, and some were older, some married and some single. They shared their experiences, their stories, their insights, and their lives with us, and we appreciate that immensely. The story of what men experience as weight loss patients has never really been studied or told, and we're proud to be one of the first to draw attention to the special needs of male bariatric patients, and bring this knowledge to the general public.

The men we talked to were not afraid to tell us that they were afraid. Some had a fear of dying from the procedure, but they also had a fear of dying without it. All but one had a fear of having a big open incision scar, and that one fellow didn't really have the fear because he was never given the option for a laparoscopic procedure by his surgeon. He was a candidate, but it was never even discussed or offered.

Others had very real fears of dealing with dumping syndrome, and strangely not one of them really had it. They also feared the procedure not working and the weight staying put. That fear was the hardest to work through before going into surgery, and most said they didn't really get rid of it until they'd lost about fifty pounds. We believe one of our interviewees, Scott, said it best: "I couldn't try it on to see if it was going to fit!"

To Scott, as to many of the other men we talked to, the fear of the drastic life change was daunting, at best. They feared not knowing what they would be able to eat (or drink!), and they feared things just being "different." It's a well known fact that men fear change more than women (as a general rule), and these men were no exception.

Almost all said they had to deal with fears about other complications as well, and for the men who had their surgeries at a non-multidisciplinary practice, the fears of complications were amplified because complications like pulmonary embolism, hernia, gallbladder disease, leaks, and obstructions were never defined nor discussed.

Having said that, not one of them expressed a fear of having a stricture or a gallbladder issue.

Two of the men we talked to did have strictures, and one had it three times, just like Julie had. He didn't have quite as bad a time with it, and he too survived the stricture fairy. One of the patients had a post-operative gallbladder issue like Karen had, for which I prescribed medication, and it resolved itself without surgical intervention. Another patient experienced a more serious complication: the bowel was not working at all for a few days after surgery, but fortunately it spontaneously resolved itself.

That was about it as far as complications went, and as for after-effects I was surprised to hear how many of these men had "scramps," to use little Meghan's word. They spoke of severe cramping in both their legs and their diaphragms/abdomens, and strangely described it exactly as Julie and Karen had described it to me months ago. Two of the patients also told us, almost sheepishly, that they had this weird sneezing response to eating heavier foods, carbohydrates, or anything that got stuck. Karen was vindicated and she let out a whoop that could be heard in south Florida!

Speaking of whoops, all of these patients were extremely happy to report that they had gone into the surgery with a variety of the most basic types of co-morbidities, and all but one man had every co-morbidity completely resolved. That one patient had five medications for high blood pressure cut back to only one. In addition to high blood pressure, these patients had high cholesterol, sleep apnea (including having it so bad as to require a machine to help breathing at night), insulin dependent diabetes, joint issues, circulation issues, back problems, and gastroesophageal reflux (chronic heartburn). All patients have seen 100% resolution of their co-morbidities, with the exception of the high blood pressure patient mentioned above. The men were more than eager and excited to detail those stories for us in the interviews.

One of the topics they were not so eager to talk about, however, was their behavior modification as it relates to food. The men all said that they still had food issues with which they grapple, and they were surprised to find that to be very normal. The biggest complaints were dealing with not drinking during meals, staying away from bad foods, chewing their food well enough, getting their water requirement in, and maintaining appropriate portion sizes. They said those things were daily struggles. The biggest one, however, was slowing down their eating. Every one of them said that was an issue on some level, and they still found themselves in "shovel" mode (eating too fast) when eating.

Other food issues included forgetting to pack food with them when they go out, and difficulty finding appropriate food and protein sources when at work or anywhere outside the home. Most of the patients confessed to being seduced on a regular basis by restaurants and fast food joints, and reported tremendous difficulties with avoiding these temptations. Luckily they also reported that the majority of the time they are able to avoid the siren call of the fast food vendors, and make good and healthy food choices.

For many men, cooking is an issue. Lots of guys just don't really know how to cook, and that's part of the reason they put on weight in the first place; pizza, fast food, restaurant food, and vending machine type snacks will do it to you every time. Some of the men we talked to knew how to cook, but rarely did. They informed us that they have taken over more of the cooking duties now (albeit mostly grilling), and that has helped with keeping up with their protein. For two others, cooking has been a newly acquired skill, and they are still attempting to master the culinary art.

We asked our patient participants about another newly acquired skill, and that was life without alcohol. One man said that he rarely drank anything anymore, maybe a small glass of wine with dinner. He said that his friends didn't like that aspect of his new life, as they used to include alcohol in many of their activities. Many others, however, said that it was really no big deal to give up drinking.

The beer drinkers either gave it up completely or switched to a non-alcoholic brew (which they found still had some effect, although greatly reduced). Yet another said he still had an occasional drink when hanging out with buddies just to keep the ribbing down to a bare minimum. He said he experienced a quicker response to the alcohol, and it gave him quite a bit of gas, but no dumping unless he drank it too fast. He said nursing one beer along through an entire football game was the way to go.

The fear of dumping, combined with the intensified effect of the alcohol was the main reason most of these men chose to avoid drinking. We were surprised to learn, however, that the second biggest reason for avoiding alcohol was the empty calories that would go primarily right to fat. It was rewarding to know that we had instilled those rationales deep enough to be applied in any food situation including situations that involve choosing or not choosing alcohol.

Several of the men reported that alcohol causes bloating, a phenomenon they never noticed when they were heavier. Many also stated that they were surprised to find that they could gain and lose between three and five pounds in water weight as well. They all said they didn't know men could carry water weight. In fact, all humans can carry water weight. When the body becomes dehydrated it attempts to conserve as much water as possible, rather than keeping it flushing through the system.

Many of the guys we spoke with also expected to have a major surge of energy immediately following surgery, or shortly thereafter. They were surprised to learn that it took a little longer than that, but eventually that surge kicked in, and now they're clicking on all cylinders. Although some of our guys were getting regular exercise, most of them reported that it was still very difficult, as they had long established patterns of inactivity that they were finding very hard to break. We were informed by one patient, and asked to remind the public at large that "not all men are genetically encoded to be sports fanatics, whether watching or playing them."

Whether they exercised or not, most of the men we talked to told us that they had lost a significant amount of weight – off their rear ends! Now I imagine that to many female readers this sounds like a very positive thing, but as we found out, it is more of a problem than we thought for male patients. The male patients who discussed losing weight off their buttocks, all recounted to us that the biggest problem is pain when sitting. It simply hurts to be sitting right on the pelvic bones. They said that the discomfort doesn't take long to set in either, and many are now avoiding situations in which they might have to sit for long periods of time.

One of the patients said that he was seriously considering getting buttock implants, not for the vanity of having a very nicely shaped butt, rather for the cushioning, and to fill out the seat of all his "baggy-butt" pants. For those of you who may be unfamiliar with "butt implants," the procedure is basically the same as the breast implant procedure, only the implants enhance the buttocks region of the body. They all stated that they were very self-conscious of their now flattened posteriors, and fitting clothes was hard enough without having to constantly have the seats of their pants taken in.

The clothing issues were a big sore spot with the majority our male interviewees as well. Several of the guys said that they still had a terrible time finding clothes to fit because of their new proportions. Men's clothes are all based on inches, and specifically men's pants are all based on waist inches and inseam inches with the waist generally being larger than the inseam. For several of these guys, however, their inseams are actually the same as, or longer than their waist sizes, and that makes pants that fit properly very hard to find.

The other issues raised about clothes included the fact that men don't generally share or trade clothes like women do, primarily because of the waist/inseam combinations, so getting clothes from a buddy isn't really an option. Other men complained of the price of replacing business clothes, and the fact that they found that suits can only be tailored down two sizes. They found that to be expensive, and said they weren't prepared for the cost. For the most part, the men did say that they would attend a clothing swap even if it meant only picking up a few smaller shirts or suits for a minimal price.

Several of the men asked Julie and Karen if they had any shopping tips on where to find clothes. Being the big-game bargain hunters that they are, they informed the men that they should be shopping at discounters and liquidators. These types of stores tend to carry unusual or off sizes, and sell at seriously discounted prices which helps the budget out a little too. Garage sales, thrift stores, and consignment shops are also good bets for very inexpensive replacement clothes, including suits and ties (remember, you'll probably have to replace the ties too as the big and tall men's ties will end up being too long).

Several of the guys told us that it was very hard to get a perspective on their new sizes as they shrank, because they would go back to the big and tall men's store, and the sales people there would, of course, sell them things. One of the men said, "The sales people still see you as a big guy, so they point you toward big clothes. I still start in the big clothes and then have to work my way down. Inevitably I end up coming out with something that is still too big, or becomes too big a week later."

We suggest a cheaper alternative: get someone to take some digital or Polaroid shots of you before you shop. Have them taken full length, and have them taken in the same spot, next to the same things every time. This will help to give you perspective, and let you see what's really there, and what really isn't anymore. It should also help you to start trying on clothes closer to your actual size.

Julie and Karen suggest that if you're still in the active shrink phase, then don't buy clothes that fit unless you are wearing it out of the store. Buy clothes a little bit snug so they'll fit longer. You'll shrink into it, have no fear. And men, there is no shame in buying goal clothing – something you hang there and shrink into. Whether it's an Armani suit or a pair of Levis you wore in high school, set some goal clothing and celebrate when you fit into it. Nobody else has to know but you.

If you have weight loss surgery, the shrinking you will so come to cherish and despise is greatly facilitated by the ingestion of your daily vitamins. We asked the guys about the pre-natal vitamin issue, and we got responses that were all over the map. The men who did not have surgery at a multi-disciplinary practice were not prescribed vitamins of any sort, and in fact, one man was told he could never take vitamins again, which is totally false and misleading.

The men who were taking vitamins did say that they had a heck of time getting their insurance companies to pay for them. For all but one, the insurance companies agreed to pay after their doctors called and explained the situation. They told us of the funny looks at the pharmacy counter when picking them up. One guy found that quite hysterical, as he said he saved himself all that embarrassment and just has his wife pick them up. She's the one who gets to deal with the funny looks.

Most of the guys admitted to skipping their vitamins about half the time, and when asked why, answered that they just felt stupid taking vitamins at all, let alone pre-natal vitamins. Two of the guys were even afraid that they might contain female hormones or something because they were "pre-natal." To be very clear, pre-natal vitamins do not contain any female hormones. They are nutritional supplements only. They augment your food intake to keep your body functioning at a better efficiency level. They are not for "wussies," nor are they unmanly. Take your vitamins! You'll have more stamina to get through the day!

Speaking of stamina, that brings us to probably the biggest issue for men in having this surgery: their sex lives. All of the men we talked to reported having a significantly improved sex drive. They stated that their sexual encounters were more sustained, more frequent, and their stamina was markedly improved. The men told us that they felt more desirable and attractive as they lost weight. As their self-images improved, so did their outlook on sex. Many said that it was much more enjoyable, varied, and not as laborious as before surgery. One man simply said, "It's not uncomfortable anymore."

The men who were in relationships told us that the weight loss had improved their view of themselves, and combined with their improved sex lives, lead to stronger and closer intimate relationships. The closer the relationships became the more communication was occurring, and the less the men found themselves withdrawing from their partners. Several of the men told us that before surgery they were just pulling away, and closing others out because of how badly they felt about themselves.

Now they report being fully committed and engaged in their relationships again, and they attribute most of that change to the change within themselves.

The changes in how they viewed themselves also affected other relationships as well. Those men with children stated that they had far more interaction with their children now, and enjoyed being able to participate in activities with them. One man, Brian, told us that it meant the world to him that his thirteen year old daughter was proud of him. We're proud of you too Brian.

Other men also told us about issues that arose with friends and relatives who were not so supportive. Karl told us that many of his friends and family were worried that he had simply taken the easy way out. They were worried that he was going to die because he so drastically cut down his eating. They unknowingly attempted to undermine his efforts out of sheer worry, fear, and lack of understanding. He said he simply wasn't prepared for that, but dealt with it appropriately.

Another man told us that he wasn't prepared for his other overweight friends to shun him because they could no longer relate to him as a result of his changed eating behaviors. On a similar note, other interviewees talked to us about how the dynamics changed with their friends because of changing size.

Apparently for several of these guys, there was an unwritten understanding that with size went proportional strength. In other words, Jeff's buddies assumed that if Jeff was "big" he must also be very strong. When Jeff began to lose weight, and despite packing on at least 20 pounds of muscle, the assumption became that Jeff was now much weaker. This assumption was confirmed for Jeff's friends when one of them went to punch him in the arm in a friendly gesture of greeting, and virtually knocked Jeff to the ground. The "old" Jeff wouldn't have budged, while the new Jeff was a push over. Jeff wasn't expecting the male friendship dynamics to change in that way. Neither were we, frankly.

In exploring that a little further, we found that increased respect for self does change the dynamics of all relationships for men, whether they be intimate, familial, social, or work related. To get to the point of self respect and increased self-esteem, the emotional work that has to be done during this process was also very unexpected to most of these men.

Like the average "Joe," most of these guys thought that they had no emotional issues with which to deal. To their profound dismay, they found that they did have some emotional baggage from years of being heavy, and it had to be unloaded along with the weight. They found that in order to ditch some of this baggage, they had to turn to the women in their lives for support, because most of their male friends were not equipped or inclined to really help.

Even in the support groups where others are struggling with similar issues, many men told us that they turned to women for help, understanding, and insight because men just don't turn to other men for emotional support. It was hard for them because they were often turning to virtually total strangers for validation of their emotional issues, and yet they could only feel comfortable turning to unfamiliar women rather than unfamiliar men. We were a bit surprised and made special note of the emotional privacy issue.

Men seemed to have an inordinate sensitivity to keeping the fact of their surgeries quite private as well. Many said they just don't tell people they had surgery "because it's none of their business." Some said that they don't tell people because of the prevailing misconception that it's the easy way out, and you're just lazy and want a quick fix. They said they get tired of defending their decisions to have surgery (we hear that a lot), so they just don't admit to it to prevent being seen as weak.

The unanimous view of these men after surgery, however, is that they are anything but weak. They are stronger, leaner, healthier, and happier now. Although they are men, their experiences are not completely dissimilar from female bariatric patients. The men told us that they all enjoyed being able to get around easier, fitting into places and things they couldn't before, and being able to participate in physical activities.

Like other weight loss surgery patients, they found it hard to go back and look at "before" pictures, they could get life insurance now where before they couldn't, and food no longer controlled them. Interestingly, several of the men said that it disturbed them deeply to watch other people eating in a restaurant as it brought up too many painful reminders of their own self-abuse with food.

These men told us that they avoid like the plague any foods that will cause dumping, and chase their protein requirements every day like an elusive fox on an English hunt. They experience no basic differences in complications or instance rates, nor are their after-effects any more concentrated in one area over another. Brian did tell us that the air in his abdomen after surgery (the beach ball effect) felt like an "internal wedgie." We thought that was pretty funny, and Karen and Julie both said it was a rather accurate statement.

Despite the possibility of a very short term internal wedgie, all of these men expressed to us that they had no regrets at all about having this surgery, including the ones who were not cared for at a multi-disciplinary practice. When asked what they would tell other men who were considering surgery, here's some of what they had to say:

"Don't do it for vanity, do it to save your life."

"Just do it. It will help in more ways than you can imagine."

"This is not the easy way out. It's hard work and sometimes frustrating, but consider what your quality of life is like right now. Could it be any worse?"

"Don't hesitate because you're a tough guy or being macho. Do it, and do it now."

"It wasn't just a lack of willpower that got you fat, so don't just rely on willpower to get it off. Get the help you need."

"Really learn about this surgery, then explain all the potential problems and benefits to your family, including your kids. Make sure they understand. Tell them in an age appropriate way. Include them in the decision process."

"Don't listen to all the media hype on the mortality rate of this surgery. Find out your own facts and don't let the media make the decision for you. They don't have your life in mind when they run those stories for ratings and advertising dollars."

"Be afraid, but do it anyway."

We couldn't have said it better ourselves! We hope that we've shed a little light on what men experience with this surgery and metamorphosis. If you're a man thinking about weight loss surgery, our advice is to talk to other men who've had the surgery, and to really discuss the subject with your doctor. Take a really hard look at the risks, benefits, alternatives, and complications of both obesity and weight loss surgery, and compare them side by side with your doctor. Make an informed decision, and whatever path you choose, make a plan to become healthy, lose the weight, and live a better quality of life. No matter the choice, here's to you finding a multi-disciplinary medical and support team who'll be behind you all the way.

Chapter Eleven

FENG SHUI
— FOR THE BODY —
AND MIND

Carrie A. Liebrock, R.D.
Scott H. Glass, M.S., M.A., L.L.P.

Hi. It's us again, Julie and Karen. We're back. We thought we needed to make an introductory statement or two for this chapter, so we're butting in on Carrie and Scott. We feel we must apologize from the start about the dog story in this chapter. It's gross, but it's funny, so we voted to keep it. Okay, with that done we'll get down to business.

We've entitled this chapter "Feng Shui for the Body and Mind" not to endorse or educate you about the ancient Chinese practice of Feng Shui (pronounced "Fung Shway"), but to use it as an analogy for taking care of the environment in which you travel through life. The reason it's such a good analogy is because the real practice of Feng Shui is about creating a healthy flow of life energy, or "chi" within the space where we spend most of our time.

We all may think that we spend most of our time at work, or at home, or maybe even in the car. But, the truth is we spend the most time (indeed all of our time) in one place: our bodies. So if we are to learn from the analogy, we must look at finding a way to create a healthy life force, or "chi" in our own bodies, and that is exactly what this chapter is about.

Feng Shui is considered a metaphysical science in which one learns to recognize and tap into the "chi" to help achieve many life endeavors. We all know that we feel better, do more, achieve more, and believe in ourselves more when we are healthy, and look and feel good about ourselves. So being healthy certainly aids us in achieving our many life endeavors.

Now, according to ancient Chinese belief, all true life changing power lies in working with the rules of nature. What more basic rule of nature is there than eating natural foods in a moderate amount for the purpose of nourishing the body, and moving the muscles of the body in such a way as to keep it running and in good working order? That's the definition of how we stay alive! What's more natural and basic than that, right?

So, by following this basic rule of nature and being healthy, it naturally follows that we will increase the life force within ourselves, feel better about ourselves, interact with the rest of the world more, and thus achieve many life endeavors.

We've examined the facts, and proven true the assertion that "life changing power lies in working with the rules of nature." If we eat healthy, and live in a healthy body, other things in our lives work out a little better for us too. Okay! Is it that easy? No. So, let's move on to the next step.

The ancient tradition is also about following the rules of nature, and about finding some harmony between all the varying elements of your life. So what are we trying to harmonize? Well, we're trying to harmonize health, good nutrition, movement, sensory satisfaction, variety, and minimize pain, discomfort, and distaste. That's just the attempt at "harmonizing" your mind is making regarding food choices and eating properly, as well as in trying to get your carcass off the couch to move for five minutes! You are constantly "assessing" all the options, and trying to "harmonize" the options to create the best possible, least offensive outcome for yourself.

Feng Shui is also considered to be the art of "assessing." It is about "assessing" quality of life through observations and analysis of a person's living environment. Again, we come back to the fact that your primary living environment is your body. As overweight people, we know far too well that the quality of your life is dictated by your weight and self-esteem, both of which are part of your primary living environment – your body. So we must assess through observation and analysis how to change the primary living environment in order to positively affect the life force within, and the quality of life we seek. Okay. So how do you do that? Glad you asked.

The first step taken in Feng Shui is to change the living environment. (We're usually talking about your house here.) This step is called "space clearing." "Space clearing" is defined as a technique that will cleanse your living environment of the negative energy that naturally accumulates over time. Well I don't know about you, but our bodies and lives have certainly accumulated some "negative energy" over time in the form of poor self-esteem, extra pounds, and emotional baggage from both. So by choosing to lose weight, you're starting your space clearing right off the bat.

To properly perform your space clearing, you'll need the help of a behaviorist (emotional and habit cleaning), a dietitian and an exercise physiologist (extra pounds and self-esteem cleaning). You will deal with and dispose of much of the emotional baggage and bad habits, and will learn to take care of your primary living environment in a natural and healthy way. In so doing, many (but not all) of the other issues and difficulties in your life may seem to clear away, or at least become more manageable.

Feng Shui theorizes that by combining space clearing with the elimination of unnecessary clutter, and a commitment to keeping your living environment as clean and functional as possible, you can begin to make real and lasting changes in your life. We wholeheartedly agree with this theory.

This chapter will provide you with many of the tools to make real and lasting changes in your life, even if you don't choose to have surgery. It's not the same old tired speech you've heard about the food pyramid, and exercising until you drop. We think you'll be pleasantly surprised at the information and advice Carrie and Scott are going to give you. So read on. You'll be glad you did.

And again, sorry about the dog part, but we're still laughing. Take it away, Carrie.

THE CARE AND FEEDING OF YOUR "CHI"

Hi. I'm Carrie Liebrock, the registered dietitian they nabbed for this project. Though my family will often lovingly refer to me as the "food police" when I attempt to lovingly encourage them to eat a little healthier, I can assure you that I have never attended any sort of food policing academy, nor is it my goal in life to incriminate those for what they choose to eat. The reason that I chose to major in dietetics rather than criminal justice was to in some way help everyone I meet become a little healthier. I just wasn't feeling that vibe in criminal justice. Call me crazy, but I prefer non-violent client interaction, and an office, not a jail cell to work in. It's a personal thing.

As a dietitian working with weight loss patients, I've heard it all when the office door closes. There have been confessions of "cheating," frustrations about weight not lost, stories of foods not tolerated, and expressions of anger, happiness, sadness, disappointment, excitement, anxiety, laughter, and even tears (sound familiar, Julie?).

You name it, I've heard it! At times I've even thought of asking the patient if perhaps their appointment was supposed to be with the behaviorist not the dietitian. But, with all of that said, I wouldn't trade what I do for anything, because helping people through those times, good, bad, or as ugly as they might be, is incredibly rewarding for me. Although I work pretty hard, I only wish I could work harder and do more for my patients.

Since it would be illegal, and lets face it, a little scary, to have myself cloned so that I could be a shadow to each of my patients as they leave my office, (more than one of me? Yikes!...), the next best thing I can do is educate them. So given the fact that they haven't yet invented the home cloning kit, let's begin by learning a little bit about the practical side of nutrition.

We'll start with nutrients. A person's daily nutrient requirements should be met through the foods they eat when possible. Nutrients are categorized into two different groups: macronutrients and micronutrients. Macronutrients include carbohydrates, protein, fat, and water. Micronutrients include vitamins and minerals. First, I'll chat a bit about the micronutrients, and get them out of the way.

Micronutrients consist of vitamins and minerals. Vitamins and minerals do not contain any calories, and are ideally obtained through the foods we eat. Supplementation is often necessary, however, for bariatric patients because of the malabsorptive and/or restrictive components of the surgery. Let's think about the word supplement and what it means; it means "to add to," not replace.

Supplements add to the diet, they do not replace foods, mainly because they do not contain the macronutrients our bodies' need. I'll explain that in a minute. Additionally, folic acid, vitamin B12, iron, and calcium aren't absorbed as well following gastric bypass surgery because of the malabsorptive component, and because patients are limited in the amount of food they can eat. Many necessary micronutrients are not being absorbed in quantities adequate for the body's needs, and therefore supplementation is recommended pre and post-operatively to ensure patients get their requisite nutrients. In short: take your pre-natal vitamins!

Well, that's about it for micronutrients, so on to macronutrients. This is the stuff we generally call "food," including protein, water, fat, and carbohydrates. We'll tackle these in reverse order, starting with carbs.

Carbohydrates are the main energy source for our bodies, and they contain approximately four calories per gram. Once eaten, carbohydrates turn into glucose, which is our body's form of sugar. Eating too many carbohydrates causes excess glucose in the body, which is stored in the liver or muscles, and converted to fat. From there it is stored as nasty body fat that causes us to hate the fat, but amazingly, not the carbohydrates.

So...do carbohydrates make us fat? If eaten in excess, yes. Are carbohydrates bad? No. Repeat after me, CARBOHYDRATES ARE NOT BAD! Anything consumed in excess is not good, whether carbohydrates, cheesecake, or too much Chardonnay on a Saturday night. Too much is just not good. M-O-D-E-R-A-T-I-O-N is the key. Easier said than done, but true nonetheless. I hope all of the low-carbohydrate dieters, and carbohydrate Nazis have heard me loud and clear. I proudly proclaim: "I eat carbs!"

I like to look at foods not as good or bad, but as some being better for you than others. The better carbohydrates to choose are the complex carbohydrates, which include fruits, whole grains, legumes, and vegetables. Complex carbohydrates provide us with vitamins, minerals, fiber, and of course energy.

Fiber, incidentally, is a wondrous thing. Fiber helps to keep us fuller longer, it can lower cholesterol, keep us regular, and since our bodies have to work harder to digest it, it can also increase our metabolism. Because of this slower digestion process, carbohydrates are turned into glucose less quickly. So, what I like to tell my patients is to eat everything in its most natural state, or "closer to God and nature" as my dear dietitian friend and mentor, Bunee' Morrison likes to say.

High fiber foods sometimes "talk behind your back" as one of my patients refers to it, so proceed with caution when adding these foods back into the diet. Gas, bloating, and cramping can occur if too much fiber is consumed. On the other hand, fiber might be just what the dietitian ordered for that common constipation problem that can occur after surgery. It'll make your body do the work it is supposed to do.

Also, make your body do the work at processing the foods, rather than buying foods such as white bread, white rice, or white pasta, where the processing has already been done. These processed, refined carbohydrates turn into sugar faster in our bodies, making us hungry sooner, and they offer little nutritional value. Instead, choose whole-wheat bread, whole-wheat pasta, brown or wild rice, dried beans, fresh fruits, and vegetables.

It can often be difficult for post-surgery patients to consume carbohydrates. Many of the carbohydrate containing foods, i.e., breads, rice, and noodles, are often hard for patients to tolerate. They can swell up, and become gummy if not processed, prepared, or cooked well. Patients complain that they sit heavy, and often there isn't room for them after eating the protein first.

In contrast, however, be aware that other carbohydrate containing foods, such as crackers, chips, corn chips, and the like seem to go down just fine for most patients that I see. These foods are crunchy, and can be chewed to a very fine consistency with no problem. Unfortunately, they are usually of low nutritive value, so limit your intake of these foods. That brings us now to simple carbs.

Sweets are considered simple carbohydrates. Foods such as fruit, milk, and yogurt contain natural sugars, and are good for you. Cakes, candies, cookies, and ice cream are processed sugars that are high in calories, and usually fat. They are not good for you. In addition, sweets can sometimes cause "dumping syndrome" after surgery.

Do not in any way, however, count on surgery or "dumping syndrome" as your sweet tooth cure, because some patients are able to tolerate sweets after surgery. On the other hand, some patients completely lose their desire for sweets of any kind. Most patients that I see can tolerate a small amount (meaning one cookie, not three), on occasion. Those that push the envelope usually end up on "auto eject," and running for the restroom.

Avoiding sweets all together would be best, although maybe not realistic. Keep in mind that sugar-free does not mean calorie-free, and some sugar-free foods contain sugar alcohols, a derivative of sugar that when eaten in excess can cause gas, bloating, and diarrhea. So, even though we want you to get lots of exercise, running to the bathroom is not what we had in mind, and I'm sure not what you had in mind either. Well, that's about all for carbs, so on to fat.

Fat offers nine calories per gram. The word "fat" has a negative connotation to it, some of which is warranted, but let's not forget that it is an important nutrient that our bodies require. Fat is a source of energy, it's our body's insulation, it regulates hormones, and it protects our organs from injury. Fat aids in the absorption of certain vitamins such as vitamins A, D, E, and K. It adds flavor and texture to foods, and since it is the last to be digested, it keeps us fuller, longer.

Too much fat obviously makes us fat, and it can lead to heart disease; and that brings us back to that word "moderation" again. The amount of fat a person should have in their diet varies depending upon age, gender, height, and weight. For successful weight loss, bariatric patients should typically try to limit their overall fat intake to less than thirty grams of fat per day.

The majority of fat in the diet should come from monounsaturated fat sources. These foods are generally liquid at room temperature, and come from plant or vegetable origins such as olive or canola oil, avocados, natural peanut butter, nuts, and olives. The monounsaturated fats help to lower our bad cholesterol (LDL cholesterol), and raise our good cholesterol (HDL cholesterol). This good cholesterol helps to clean out the bad cholesterol in our bodies, so having a higher HDL level is important.

Another type of fat, polyunsaturated fat also comes from plant or vegetable origins such as safflower or sunflower oil, and some seeds and nuts. Though these foods help to lower overall cholesterol, they do tend to lower the HDL cholesterol as well. Eating less polyunsaturated fat, and more monounsaturated fat is advised.

Polyunsaturated Omega 3 fats, however, are considered good fats. These are found in deep ocean fish, such as salmon and tuna, as well as nuts, flaxseed, and flaxseed oil. These fats are often referred to as "brain fats." They help to lower triglycerides, prevent stroke, and in some studies have been shown to help with depression.

The bad guys, or saturated fats, are generally solid at room temperature, and come from animal sources such as bacon, butter, lard, ice cream, 2% and whole milk, regular cheese, and regular sour cream. Saturated fats raise our cholesterol, and clog our arteries putting us at risk for heart disease.

Our bodies need almost no saturated fats, so limit the intake of these foods. Unless you are under the age of two, in need of gaining weight, or are a baby cow, there is no need to be drinking 2% or whole milk. Instead, choose 1%, ½%, skim, or soymilk. Choose low fat cheeses, and low fat sour cream instead of the regular, full fat version to help limit your saturated fat intake.

Worse than saturated fats, however, are hydrogenated fats or trans fats. Once a "hidden" fat found in foods such as crackers and many low fat snacks and sweets, trans fats are now being listed on the nutrition facts food labels. And thanks goodness, as hydrogenated or trans fats are pesky little fat-makers.

Hydrogenation is a chemical process in which foods are made more solid (like saturated fats), giving them the texture and taste many Americans like. Hydrogenation also aids in food preservation, allowing foods to sit on the shelf for as long as year. So, again, I will remind you to eat foods in their most natural state, not a chemically made state. If the ingredient list is as long as this chapter, it cannot be good for you.

In addition to processed foods, the bariatric patient should avoid fatty, greasy, and fried foods. Though I like a french fry as much as the next person (especially if it has cheese all over it), fried foods eaten in excess make all of us gain weight. Because fat stays in our stomachs the longest, and is the last to be digested, it can cause acid reflux, and nobody likes that.

Cramping, bloating, and diarrhea, or "dumping syndrome" can also occur if the patient consumes these types of foods. I've had patients who removed the breading from fried fish before eating it, and still became ill from the grease that had seeped through to the meat of the fish. So, be careful, and ask yourself: will those foods help me to lose weight? No. So why eat them? Have a glass of water instead.

Ahh, water. Can anything be more natural? How fabulous can it be? It has no calories, suppresses the appetite, hydrates us, helps to breakdown fat, relieves fluid retention, helps maintain muscle tone, flushes waste and toxins out of our bodies, and helps keep us regular. What more do you need?

Bariatric patients should consume a minimum of sixty-four ounces of non-carbonated, diet, caffeine-free fluids per day. Water is the best choice. If you don't recall why it's the best choice re-read the previous paragraph. If patients don't want to consume all sixty-four ounces as water, they should absolutely consume at least half, or thirty-two ounces as water. An avid water drinker myself (at least sixty-four ounces per day), I highly recommend and encourage my patients to drink all sixty-four ounces as water.

Patients should avoid drinking with their meals following surgery, as this can cause nausea and vomiting. Not only does it cause nausea and vomiting, it washes food out of the pouch twice as fast. Patients then lose some of the protein they ate, and they become hungry sooner. If patients do not avoid drinking with their meals, or do not wait to drink for an extended period of time after meals, they increase their chances for weight gain after surgery. That's a scary thought.

More water is also needed if patients are suffering from vomiting, diarrhea, and/or constipation. If you're experiencing one of these things, sucking down a glass of water is generally not the first thing on your mind, but it will help. Vomiting and diarrhea deplete the body's supply of water, and constipation is caused in part by a lack of it. Hydrating the body helps all the way around.

It is imperative that patients keep themselves hydrated before and after surgery, and avoiding caffeine is one way to do that. Because caffeine is a diuretic it can dehydrate us, which, hello! is the exact opposite of what we want!

Caffeine is also a gastric stimulant and can make us hungrier – just what you want when you are trying to lose weight, right? Wrong! Caffeine, along with some acids (like those in soda pop), also leach calcium from our bones, which can cause osteoporosis down the road. When you consider that calcium is not absorbed as efficiently after weight loss surgery, don't add insult to injury by consuming caffeine or soda pop.

Speaking of pop, carbonation can be painful and bloat patients after surgery. If you have stopped drinking caffeine and carbonated beverages before surgery, by all means do not return to consuming them after surgery.

Our society drinks way too much pop as it is. This includes all kinds of pop, including the clear ones. The acid in pop is just barely below lethal. With every mouthful, it so drastically alters the pH level of your body that your body then has to cough up some hard mineral to balance it out again in order to keep you breathing. The first thing it coughs up is calcium (which you are having a hard time getting enough of to begin with!), and it gets it directly from your bones.

Don't believe me? Do some research on the web. Many physicians have written about the dangers of soda pop. There is nothing good for you in pop, unless of course you think all those chemicals in pop are preserving you somehow for the next century! Chemicals and sugar are the least of your worries. In fact, if you're a weight loss surgery patient, the carbonation will probably get you before anything else will. I refer you again to Julie and Karen's treatise on air bubbles in Chapter Four.

Soda pop causes dehydration, and another thing that can cause dehydration after surgery is alcohol. I will again say that if you did not consume alcohol prior to surgery, please do not start after. Alcohol provides seven "empty" calories per gram. They're empty because there is no nutritional value to alcohol, and for bariatric surgery patients it causes other problems as well.

After surgery alcohol passes through the new pouch directly into the second portion of the small bowel, known as the jejunum. The jejunum has a large surface area that readily and rapidly absorbs the alcohol, making patients "cheap drunks" after surgery. I believe Julie has already related to you her experience with alcohol. If I had a nickel for every time I heard one of those stories…. As you can see, bottled, or even tap water is the way to go. So drink up, and drink plenty!

The last macronutrient that I want to talk about is protein. The reason I saved protein for last is because it is probably the most important nutrient that the bariatric patient can consume. Protein provides four calories per gram, and it is the basic structural material of all cells. It helps to build and repair new tissues, aids in wound healing, provides satiety, prevents hair loss, and it preserves muscle tissue. Protein gives red blood cells their structure, and it helps antibodies function properly. It also helps in the regulation of enzymes and hormones.

Protein chains are created through a combination of amino acids, most of which we should be getting from our food sources. Amino acids are the building blocks of protein, and they are either "essential," or "non-essential." Our body makes the non-essential amino acids we need, but the essential amino acids must come from the foods we eat.

Essential amino acids found in the proteins we eat are either "complete," or "incomplete." The complete proteins, also known as "high biological value" proteins, come primarily from animal sources, and they contain all nine essential amino acids that our bodies need. Cheese, meat, eggs, milk, yogurt, and soy are examples of these.

Incomplete proteins, such as beans, grains, nuts, and vegetables, lack one or more of the essential amino acids. Therefore, two incomplete proteins, or an incomplete and complete protein must be combined to make the protein more useful to the body. An example would be beans and rice. Together they make a complete protein, but they don't necessarily have to be eaten at the same meal.

For patients, protein is emphasized right from the start. Approximately two weeks prior to surgery patients are put on a high protein diet, which should not be confused with some of those popular high protein, low carbohydrate, high fat diets out there. Having been vegetarian for nearly thirteen years now, I'm certainly not an advocate of the Atkins® diet, and in fact, would love to de-Atkinize most of the world. But, I will jump off my anti-Atkins® soapbox and move on….

Patients are generally placed on a high protein "fast" prior to surgery. "Fast," meaning patients are starved before surgery? Heavens no. Though the term "fast" does mean to abstain from food, we do not starve our patients. Patients may feel as though they are starving, considering what most were eating prior to the fast, but they do survive (is that Gloria Gaynor I hear??). What we are aiming for is to nutritionally prepare the patient for surgery as Dr. Baker stated in Chapter Three.

Patients are generally placed on a two-week supplemented fast prior to surgery, during which they consume specially formulated, high protein products that contain little sugar or fat, and are low in calories. The protein fast is approximately eight hundred calories per day, and anywhere from seventy-five, to one hundred and fifty grams of protein per day. I've had patients tell me that some of the medical protein products they've taken on medical programs in other physician's offices taste like something you'd eat on Fear Factor®. Ours don't taste that bad, and the majority of people can handle it. I suggest checking with the dietitian in your surgeon's office for more information on the products they use, what they taste like, and the related nutritional values.

After surgery, patients are generally on liquid protein anywhere from two to four weeks, and Julie and Karen have told you a little bit about that. The next step is transitioning to soft foods, such as low fat cottage cheese, cream soups made with milk, sugar-free pudding, soft eggs, deli meats, and low fat cheeses.

Patients look forward to seeing the dietitian on this day. In fact, this is usually the day that I love my job most. I'm no longer the food police. I'm no longer that "thin, mean, food lady." I am the patient's best friend. I've even had patients profess their love for me at this visit!

As you can tell, patients are usually more than ready to transition at this point. Some have even tried to eat the fake food models on my desk! And, Julie's right, they are pathetic! I've had patients tell me that their cat was even starting to look good to them! Poor Kitty! But, as you read in Chapter Six, and will read about in a different context in the following chapter, getting enough protein in after surgery can be somewhat of a challenge for patients.

One reason is that patients generally do not feel hungry again until three to six months after surgery. Therefore, patients often have to force themselves to eat after surgery, which is a concept hard to imagine for most people. I tell my patients to think of eating their protein like medicine, you have to get it in if you want to heal, if you like your hair, if you want to preserve your muscles, and if you want to have optimal weight loss. So, unless you want to be bald, skinny, flabby, and have a lot of atrophy, I suggest getting the protein in whatever way you can!

Another reason it can be challenging to get in the necessary protein after surgery is the size of the new stomach, or "pouch." It is approximately one to two ounces after surgery. Not a lot of room. So, patients have to eat small, frequent meals in order to get in all of their protein. Ideally, we'd like to see sixty or more grams of protein a day for patients, but it's often difficult for them to get in the minimum of fifty that we recommend.

After patients have been on the soft protein choices for a few weeks, they then gradually advance to more solid foods, such as meats, fruit, grains, and nuts. Because of their "roughage," raw veggies and salads are last to be added back to the diet. Patients who follow the lists given to them, do not transition themselves early to foods, follow the rules of the "pouch" tool, and get some form of exercise, will be the most successful.

Living on protein drinks and protein products after surgery is not recommended if patients are able to eat regular foods. When hunger returns you want to fill the pouch with good quality, solid foods so that you stay full for as long as you can.

Protein drinks, or any liquids with calories such as milk, juice, and thin soups go through the pouch twice as fast, slowing weight loss, and in some cases, causing weight gain. Protein supplements should only be used in cases where patients are having a difficult time getting all of their protein in natural sources.

Protein bars, which are more solid than protein drinks, are an acceptable snack after surgery. Beware though, that many of the protein bars on the market are practically glorified candy bars. Look for protein bars that are two hundred calories or less, contain less than ten grams of fat, and at least ten grams of protein per serving. Too much sugar means it tastes yummy, but you might end up in the bathroom in auto eject mode.

The most common dietary complications seen after surgery are nausea and vomiting. If patients eat too fast, if they drink while they eat, if they don't chew their food well enough, or if they eat more than their pouch can comfortably hold, they can get sick. The surgical "tool" is designed to restrict the amount of food a patient can eat. Old habits die hard, however, and just about every patient gets sick at least once.

In fact, I've heard more than I ever cared to about patients vomiting. I've heard about dry heaves. I've heard about the gagging. I've heard about the color, the consistency, and the texture of their vomit. I've even heard about a patient getting sick outside, and the dog eating it! Heck, I've even had a patient vomit in my office! It comes with the territory, and at this point, nothing phases me.

My point is, many patients learn the hard way. And, if you were a fast eater prior to surgery, you will likely be one of those that learn the hard way because you just have to slow down. Food should be chewed twenty or twenty-five times before swallowing, and patients should take thirty to forty-five minutes to eat each of their meals. If not, your dog could be in for something he didn't count on for dinner....

While we are on the subject, let's talk about pets for a minute. Because patients cannot eat the quantities they used to, I'm told by many of my patients that their pets are being fattened up with what is left on the plates, otherwise they are cooking for two: themselves and the garbage disposal. Being the animal lover that I am, I cringe at all these scraps being given to pets, and can't help but envision gastric bypass for animals in the near future.

Please don't feed all your extra food to your pets. Learn to cook smaller portions, or get some plastic food saver tubs. You know how bad you feel physically as an overweight person? They can get all the same aches, pains, and related health conditions you can, only they can't choose to lose the weight. For all those overweight pets out there, I just hope their owners are becoming more active, and taking them on more walks....

Well, I hope you have learned a little about weight loss surgery and nutrition after reading this, and that you don't feed the junk you shouldn't eat to your pet. Keep in mind that surgery is not a miracle cure, and you have to truly be ready to change your old behaviors into new behaviors.

The surgeon will do his job, the behaviorist will do his or her job, and the dietitian will do her job, but unless you do your part, the surgery will only be another failed diet attempt. We are here to help you, and to give you the tools you need to be successful; it's up to you to use these tools to their maximum potential. We know you can. You're worth it.

Now I'll hand you over to Scott who's going to make you get up and walk around while you read this part of the chapter.

Hello. It's Scott Glass again. You're friendly neighborhood behaviorist/exercise physiologist from Chapter Seven, remember? Good. Nice to see you again too. Now, we've let you avoid it as long as we can, but I promise I'll make this information as painless as possible. If you would rather clean your bathroom than exercise, you are not alone. I'm hoping to change your mindset on that. I'll bet I can, so take a deep breath and stay with me.

For many overweight people, exercise represents more aches and pains, more discouragement, more discomfort, more awkwardness, more social rejection, and more self-loathing. Who in their right mind would go out of their way for more pain? I hope that by the time you get to the end of this chapter, your attitude toward exercise will shift, even just a little. So forge ahead and keep an open mind. I believe you will find that exercise, or "movement" is not as bad as you think, and yes, you can do it.

As patients with serious weight issues, we know that your excess weight results in muscle soreness and joint pain. We know you become short of breath quickly. We understand that you are not in good physical condition. We empathize with your discouragement and hopelessness from failed exercise attempts in the past, so we are not asking you to do very much. Are you doing okay so far? Read on, it gets better!

There are three dimensions, if you will, that exercise physiologists consider when writing or evaluating an exercise plan. It helps to use an acronym, F.I.T. (Hey, at least it's not F.A.T.)

"F" is for frequency, or the number of times you do an activity in a given week. Do you walk several days a week? Ride the bike three days a week? Go get the mail everyday?

"I" is for intensity, or how hard you push yourself while doing that activity. With walking, the intensity would be your walking speed. With stationary bicycle riding, the intensity is your pedaling speed and the tension at which you have your bicycle set. With weight training, the intensity is the amount of weight you are lifting.

"T" is for time. How long, or how many minutes you do that activity each session constitutes your time interval.

If you have not had weight loss surgery yet, the most important dimension for you is frequency. Neither intensity, nor length of time is important for you right now. Although your mind may tell you to push yourself harder or longer, your body cannot handle that kind of physical stress at this point. That is what the surgery is for: to help you lose the excess body weight resulting in less stress on your muscles and joints, so you will not be so quickly short of breath, and so that you will be able to enjoy more strenuous activity. The most important goal for you at this point is for you to get into a pattern of daily activity.

Developing a healthy habit and changing your style of living requires repetition — doing it over and over, repeatedly and consistently. Remember, it doesn't have to be a lot. Just do some form of physical activity, or movement, over and above your normal daily activity, a minimum of four days per week. If you can do it five or six days a week, that would be even better. Setting your goal at seven days per week is probably unrealistic, and may result in frustration, more discouragement, and ultimately fizzling out. Don't worry yet about how long you have to do this "onerous" thing, I'll get to that in just a minute.

Thirty minutes of aerobic exercise is the medical recommendation for healthy living. Starting at 30 minutes, however, is not realistic for many people. Many patients have difficulty walking from one bench to the next bench in the mall, and are unable to walk for five minutes, let alone thirty! These people see one half hour of continuous walking as out of reach. It seems like too much. It's just not something they're able to do, and once again, they are defeated before they start.

Instead, wouldn't it be a lot easier to simply start where you already are? The main reason people fizzle out on their exercise program is most often due to starting out far too fast. After their first walk or work out, they drag themselves into their easy chair and lament, "You've got to be kidding?! Do I need to do this again tomorrow?" This person is already defeated in their attitude after their first day of moving or working out.

Contrast this with another scenario. You go for a short, leisurely walk, and you stop when you get short of breath or your knees start to ache. You have a little pep in your step, and you feel good that you did it. You say to yourself, "That wasn't too bad. I can do this again tomorrow!"

The best, and safest way to start is slow and easy. Don't push it. If you were training for a competition of some sort, a beauty contest or an athletic event, you would really need to push yourself to be ready to go by a certain date. But, we are not in any contest. Weight management is not a competition. There is no end date. There's no deadline. Weight management is a process; it is a style of living.

As you improve your style of living, the weight will come off, and as you maintain your new, healthier style of living, you will maintain your weight loss. So there is no hurry here. It is a life-long process. Get rid of all those old notions, and listen to what I'm telling you now. To quote Hans and Franz from that Saturday night show, "hear me now, and believe me later! We're here to pump (clap!) you up!

Eating less and exercising more until you reached your goal weight, was the old mindset of dieting that we are trying to get away from. It doesn't work, right? You end up gaining all the weight back and then some. Just start with small changes, one at a time. These should be changes that are small enough to make you feel confident, and to help you be consistent for the long-term.

Begin with any physical activity that will get your heart rate up and do it only as long as you are comfortable. If you decide to begin walking, and you get short of breath after 15 minutes of leisurely walking, STOP. Call it good. Do not push yourself.

You will be thinking that you should really walk further than this. You will be thinking that you could do so much more when you were younger, but that was the past, and many pounds ago. Don't allow guilt or shame to make you do more than you are able. Do what you can, and the rest will follow.

A little bit each day is the key. I would rather have a person walk for five minutes, five days per week, than have them walk one half hour once on the weekend. Even though this works out to 25 minutes compared with 30 minutes, it is the repetition that will prove to be most effective in the long run.

Give it two to three, even four weeks to get comfortable, and then bump up your time a little bit. Don't feel compelled to increase your time by ten, or even five minutes. If you feel comfortable with a two or three minute increase every other week, that would be fantastic! Remember, you are not in a race, and there is no pressure. You have the rest of your life to get your movement program where you want it. This is about life style.

There are many who will read this chapter who cannot walk for two minutes due to severe muscle weakness, severe joint pain, or excessive weight. Just do what you can. We're behind you, and we understand. I have a patient who is nearly 700 pounds, and he spends most of the day in bed. Getting out of bed is too much for him. He still has a positive attitude though, evidenced by the fact that he does leg lifts, and arm exercises in bed. We're okay with that. It's a start, and it's what he can do, and do consistently.

Many patients will start by standing up at each television commercial, walking to the kitchen, getting a drink of water, and sitting back down again. Some will simply walk in place when commercials come on. You don't have to lift your feet high, just move.

Another woman was walking the length of her ten-foot hallway in her one-bedroom efficiency apartment four times a day, over and above her normal daily activity. Don't do more than you should, but don't do less than you can either. As you lose weight and become more fit, you can do more, and you should. Worry about it when that time gets here.

Getting more physical activity is as much an attitude, as it is an activity. Do you like the direction your weight and health are going right now? If you picked up this book, probably not. Are there important things you are missing out on due to your weight? If so, then there are no alternatives. You must get up and move.

One lady stands in her kitchen leaning on the counter with stiff arms so the counter bears much of her weight, and does leg swings to the side and to the back. It's not a lot, but she has started! She is doing a little bit every day, and SO CAN YOU!

When you begin moving, and you don't set yourself up for failure by expecting to do more than your reasonably can, you will develop a better attitude about yourself, and see yourself as more in control of the situation. You will feel less like a victim. Exercise and movement have a very positive effect on attitude, self-esteem, self-worth, and overall emotional health. Everyone on the planet can benefit from movement of some sort.

Yes, everyone! Even those who have physical disabilities. There are many exercise physiologists and physical therapists who specialize in patients with disabilities. Julie had disabilities from her car accident. She had a terrible time just walking to get from one place to another, let alone walking for exercise. We sat down with her, and we found various "movements" she could do as she lost weight, and became physically stronger. Now she's walking all over the place, and we can't keep up with her! We've created a monster!

Don't worry if you have physical limitations. We understand that. We can work with it, or around it. The important thing to know is that you can do it, and it doesn't have to be painful or "onerous." As you lose the weight, your body will react differently, and your weight loss surgeon's office will have an exercise physiologist there to make sure that your movement program is keeping up with your new capabilities. It shouldn't be designed to push you, but it should be designed to determine what you are capable of doing, and therefore should be doing. Don't resist the change. Call it "progress."

Movement doesn't have to be boring either. You'll be shocked at what fun things we can come up with, and still call it exercise! Virtually any movement has some benefit to it. So, if you can add a few more sustained movements in every day, you're well on your way to creating a better and healthier life. Just don't forget to rest.

Rest is very important, and incidentally plays a vital role in weight gain and loss. The body needs to revitalize itself as much as it needs to move. That's how we are designed, and since we really can't do too much about redesigning our genetic blueprint, we just have to go with that. So move when you can and how you can, drink plenty of water, and get your sleep. That's my professional recommendation. So let's get started!

No one else has the ability to get you up and moving. So, what are you going to do? You must take responsibility and ownership for your condition. You can begin to change the direction things have been going. You can do it! It is not too late! You are valuable! You are significant and important! You are loved! You are worth it!

Whether or not you decide to have weight loss surgery, please take the first step, no matter how small, toward a healthier life. Remember: every wondrous journey begins with just one step. Stand up and take yours.

Chapter Twelve

━ THE PROTEIN SAFARI ━

Julie M. Janeway
Karen J. Sparks

Ah, Protein! The building block of life! By now, we hope you've read the previous chapter, and you've learned all about how important protein is to your body, and your life. We're not going to re-iterate that information here, but what we are going to do is discuss the many facets of living a life in search of protein.

We have named this daily quest the protein "safari," rather than the protein hunt, the protein pursuit, or the protein chase, because "safari" says it best: the adventure of hunting big-game!!

Every day is an adventure too! What you ate yesterday, may not sit well today. Your busy schedule may take you to places that give you limited opportunities to find protein, or limited time to eat. No two days are ever the same. The only constant is that you must continue to get the protein in whatever way you can.

Getting enough protein, however, is often the problem. As we've mentioned several times in this book, when you come home from the hospital you simply don't feel like putting anything in your "stomach." That's generally true no matter what type of surgery you might have (and trust me, I am a living expert on surgeries after 23 of them!) Despite the natural inclination not to eat, "if at first you don't eat, try, try again."

When I had the stricture, I couldn't get anything in. I was in bad shape. My nurse friend Judy was determined, however, to find me something I could tolerate because she knows the importance of getting enough protein every day. Judy left the college one day (basically because I looked so bad and could barely hold my head up), and came back about an hour later with $50.00 worth of protein drinks from the health food store.

What she brought helped to save my life. She bought me a product called Isopure Sport® made by a company named Nature's Best out of New York. This is a water based whey protein drink (as opposed to milk or juice based), and a 16 oz bottle contains 15 grams of protein. It is aspartame® and preservative free, and comes in fruit punch, grape, lime, mango, orange, and blue raspberry flavors. It is available with carbohydrates or without, and if you're in the position that you need this to keep you going, the carbs aren't a bad idea.

Now it's not exactly Kool-Aid®, but then it's not supposed to be. It tastes just fine if you're not expecting it to taste like something else like pop or another flavored type of drink. It is generally designed to be a nutritional supplement, but for me it was the difference between survival and dehydration. If you find yourself with a stricture, or after surgery you become intolerant of the protein products from your surgeon's office (and some people experience this), then give Isopure Sport® a try. It was a life-saver for both Karen and me when we couldn't get the protein we required to thrive and keep our hair in our heads!

You must make eating the requisite amount of protein one of the most important things you do each day. Now, we'd be lying if we said that either one of us managed to get all of our protein in every day. In fact, even when you've given it your best try, there are days that you simply don't get anywhere near your goal.

Being tired or stressed will certainly affect your ability to get and keep food in at all. Your body just seems to reject food because it doesn't want to waste the energy processing it. I guess all your energy must be going to keeping you awake, or keep you from throwing yourself off a bridge, depending on your sleep deprivation or stress load.

Speaking of being stressed, or stressing others as the case may be, diminished protein levels also affect your hormones (men have them too!) which can make you one cranky baby! Take pity on those around you, and don't purposefully turn yourself into a psychotic hormone-ravaged lunatic by perpetually evading your protein needs. We can't tell you what to do about any other hormone issues you might have, but just don't add to the problem by missing your protein.

When you do eat, you will learn to eat the protein first. Sounds simple enough, right? Wrong! You've spent a lifetime going for the starches and carbs first, and using the meat or other protein based foods simply to stuff the other food down to make more room! A lifetime habit like that doesn't go away over night.

But, you will learn to eat the protein first because after you've eaten the potatoes or the veggies, or even some salad, and you find there's simply no room left for the chicken or the fish, you figure out that you probably should have eaten the protein first. It's just like a safari: you aim, you shoot, and you miss. But, the more you aim and shoot, the more likely it is that you will eventually hit something. It just takes some people longer to learn to hit the target.

In case you're one of these slow learners, this means that you may not be figuring out that you need the protein to go in before the other foods until something drastic happens, like your hair begins to fall out. That will most certainly get your attention, and tell you to put down the fork, and step away from the potatoes.

Putting down the potatoes or veggies in favor of the meat or fish will help with something else as well: getting your protein in bigger doses. When you eat the non-protein foods first, you fill your pouch/stomach and leave less room for protein. When you are full, you're full, and you must now wait at least four to five more hours to eat again. But now you've got yourself worried that you are behind in getting that all important 50-60 grams of protein in for the day. So what happens? You graze.

Grazing means that you try to make it up in between meals with a little protein here, and a little there; but grazing leads to more calories, and a reinforcement of your previous eating habits. Grazing is not good because it is generally contrary to what your behaviorist, doctor, and dietitian are trying to help you learn. When you eat you should try to eat your protein in big doses (10-20 grams at a time). It sounds like it would be a huge amount of meat, fish, or what-have-you, but really it isn't. It's just about the size of the palm of your hand.

Eating your 10-20 grams per meal doesn't mean you can't have the other foods too. In fact, you should be learning to eat balanced meals, and if you skip the veggies too much, you'll begin to sort of crave them. But you should base the meal around the protein, which means learning to read labels and memorize protein values to determine how much protein, fat, and carbs you're combining in a meal.

It's not really a conscious thing, you just kind of start doing it. You don't really want to waste what little room you have in there on foods that don't get you where you need to go as far as your daily required intake. After a while, you'll be reading food labels as closely as a prenuptial agreement! Once you start doing this, you'll find protein in a number of unexpected places, and your meals won't just consist of a chicken breast (20-30 grams depending on size), a scoop of veggies (1-2 grams depending on veggie), and maybe a small spoonful of potatoes. Soon you'll be having wonderful meals, and your family will love them too. To get you started, visit our web site for a nifty list of protein sources Carrie threw together, and some yummy high protein recipes too!

There are many high-protein oriented cookbooks on the market, and even a number of cookbooks for people who've had weight loss surgery. I, however, do not like to cook, and never have liked to cook. I can do it when necessary, but I don't enjoy it. To me cookbooks and cooking are only useful if I'm having a party and have to lull people into thinking I'm really a Susie-homemaker. I cook only when I feel guilty because my husband is on his eighth PB&J in two days, or because I spent too much money shopping. Hate it! Hate it! Hate it!!!

Karen loves to cook, but she's single (men reading this take note!), and forever on the go. Both of us have had to learn some tricks, and learn to adapt our lives in order to get our protein every day, and thus keep our hair and lose our fat. The first of these tricks is learning to dismantle food.

If you must eat out, whether at a restaurant, someone else's house, or even the cafeteria at work, then learn to dismantle food. Look first for items that have a probable high protein content, and then look to see if things can be left off, or taken off in order to lower the calories, fat, carbs, and most of all bulk of the food. An example is a grilled chicken sandwich. You can ditch the bun, leave off the sauce or mayo, eat the lettuce and tomato, and if it needs a little something, dip it in a spot of regular mustard. That's dismantling your food.

If you're at someone's home for dinner, then skip the rolls, leave the gravy off the meat, or pick out what you can eat from the casserole. If you let someone know ahead of time that it's not their cooking, that you simply have a limited range of foods you can eat, people generally aren't offended. If you don't tell them, however, they tend to think it must be something they did, or maybe you're just rude or ungrateful.

If you're not comfortable with telling someone that you've had weight loss surgery and can only eat certain foods, and a small amount of food at that, there are other ways you can get around this. I've often quietly told people that I have food allergies, or a gastrointestinal disorder that prevents me from eating many foods.

There are many such disorders that exist, like Celiac disease, or a carbohydrate malabsorption disorder. You don't have to name what disorder you're claiming to have, simply know that many types exist that cause all kinds of people to have food issues similar to yours. It's really not all that uncommon.

The moral of the story here is: do whatever you have to do to effectively dismantle food when you're in situations that don't afford you control over what's offered or available to eat.

Second to dismantling is substituting. If you go to restaurants like Bennigans® or TGIFridays® you'll find protein friendly menu items. The problem is they often sell them with a side of broccoli. That sounds all well and good, especially if you like broccoli, but I suspect you might find that broccoli gives you terrible gas and air bubble problems. Not a plan.

If you tell the waitperson that you have a gastrointestinal disorder and can't tolerate broccoli, they'll generally substitute another vegetable without charge. These two restaurants will do that anyway, but that's just a little lawyer/daughter of a restauranteur tip for you for the restaurants that want to charge you for substitutions. Generally, if they think they could end up getting sued for feeding you something they are now on notice will make you sick, they'll suck up the 15 cents it may cost them in substituting the food.

The foregoing is just general information. Do not construe this as personal legal advice. This is an express disclaimer of all responsibility for liability claimed or incurred as a result of the previous statement. (Sorry — occupational hazard....)

Another tip for finding your protein if you hate to cook or don't have time, concerns what we affectionately call "plastic food." Plastic food is the high-protein, low-fat, low-carb frozen entrée made by the brand name of your choosing. Plastic food can be a lifesaver. Men: this will appeal to many of you.

First off, you have to choose the regular size ones – "hungryguy" dinners are no longer an option. If you choose the regular size ones, they are generally about the right amount of food, and they help teach you what proper portions should look like.

They'll give you some variety in your diet, and they give you a protein count that is pretty close to what it will say on the box (give or take an ounce or so of meat).

Plastic food also gives you a calorie count so you can keep track, and provides a decent balance of foods. Finally, they're portable, so almost anywhere you go you can have some reasonable protein available to eat, and they don't require cooking! Just slap it in the microwave, and you've got an edible pile of protein, and no dishes!

The portability of plastic food has helped Karen and me so much. We have crazy class schedules as professors, and add to that our consulting and presentation schedules, and we're just never near home cooking (unless I'm feeling guilty over shopping…) You simply can't live in restaurants or fast food joints. Not acceptable.

Restaurants get old so fast because the food has to be dismantled, and it costs an arm and a leg. You can only eat about a third of it, and the rest goes home to the styrofoam jungle until it rots and goes in the garbage. (My mom, who was raised in the "clean your plate, there are starving children in Africa" era, thinks that throwing away food is just awful. She calls it the pagan ritual of feeding the garbage-god.)

Karen and I got so sick of restaurants and trying to find foods we could eat, that we took to ordering one entrée (with appropriate substitutions and deletions) and sharing it. People look at us kind of funny, but it works out a lot better. Also, we figured out that sometimes sharing an appetizer is the way to go; like those little appetizer rib things. Protein filled, and not too much. Sometimes you have to ask if they can send things out without the sauce, or simply put it on the side. Dipping is okay, swimming in it is not.

Planning ahead and taking food with you becomes a skill you acquire. Karen and I have to travel to a lot to conferences and other speaking engagements. We plan what we're taking to eat, before we plan what we're taking to wear. Heck! We plan our food for the conference, before we plan what we're going to say in our presentation at the conference!

We take low-fat cheese sticks or cheese cubes, fat-free yogurt, small apples, bananas, peanuts (Karen likes them — I say yuck), deli shaved turkey breast, a few veggies, and things like that. We don't even go shopping, or to teach classes without planning and packing food now. You simply can't be caught without it; not if you want to keep losing weight, and keep your hair!

Now in an absolute emergency, you may be forced to stop at a fast food place to find your protein. Do not make this a habit!!! Weight loss surgery will have freed you from the heinous grasp of the fast food demon. Do not let it get it's sharp little claws into you again, or all this will have been for naught! Be as careful in going to fast food joints as you would be in walking near quicksand — or a trial lawyer. (I'm allowed to poke fun at my own kind….)

There are a few acceptable alternatives at some of these places, but for the most part they're off limits. If necessary, however, a *grilled* chicken breast sandwich minus bun and other stuff is okay, albeit expensive. Wendy's® 99 cent chili isn't bad, and the nutrition information can be found at the company's web site. Some of the salads at various places are good, but be very careful of the content of the salad dressings.

Does this mean you can never have even one french fry? No, it doesn't, but trust me on this, you won't be able to eat many. Again, I've suffered so you don't have to. Of course avoid all the fried foods, and the hamburgers of every type and description; you just can't get the fat out of them.

Some Asian food is okay, but beware the oils in which it is cooked as they contain a lot of fat, and may cause dumping syndrome. Some Mexican food is okay, but again beware what it has been cooked in, how spicy it might be, and watch the rice content as it will just keep expanding in your poor little pouch/stomach until you feel like you're going to pop! Basically, you just have to use your common sense, and watch your step when it comes to being on the daily protein safari.

To help you with what I sense to be your growing angst over the adventures involved in the daily protein safari, I suggest (and so will your dietitian and doctor I suspect) that you make a daily list or record of the protein you've consumed, the other foods consumed, your water intake, and the approximate fat, calorie, and carb counts for the day as well. Tracking the times you eat, and where you eat also helps to remind you what worked for you and what didn't. Eventually you'll be able to do all this in your head.

If you have one of those stressed or tired days that you just really can't eat, then write down what you did eat, and put the day behind you. Look at your protein totals for the whole week. Don't stress out over missing your goal (even if it's by a mile) on one particular day. This is a long haul, big-picture thing. Don't look at the snap shot, look at the whole roll of film.

Looking at things in the aggregate helps you to remain in control instead of letting the food issues control you. Isn't that kind of how you ended up fat in the first place? — emotional eating, boredom eating, stress eating? Oh, and don't forget "eating without awareness."

"Eating without awareness" is the phenomenon that occurred when you sat in front of the boob-tube and simply stuffed potato chip after potato chip (or substitute donut, cookie, cracker, pizza slice, etc.) into your mouth until, without even noticing, you'd finished off the entire bag or box. We all did that. Nobody gets to the point of considering weight loss surgery without having experienced "eating without awareness."

Although you've pretty much got the "eating without awareness" thing licked (no pun intended), the other food issues are still there skulking around in the back of your emotional vortex waiting to strike. Be vigilant! Lock, bolt, bar, block, barricade, impede, hinder, and blockade the door behind which these food issues prowl, and never again let them through!

Take care because they will lie in wait, ready to attack when your defenses are low. They're prone to strike right before your monthly cycle, after an argument with your spouse, while watching the Sopranos, or anytime during the entire boring basketball season. Opportunities abound….

To beat back these insidious little food assailants, I suggest taking a tip from the people who teach self-defense against sinister human assailants. (I do this and it really works!) When you feel some unexplainable need to stuff food in your mouth, and you know you shouldn't be, say firmly, or even forcefully, "NO!"

Now it doesn't work if you only say it in your head. We know this to be the case, because if it worked by saying it in your head, I wouldn't be writing this book, and you wouldn't be reading it. You have to actually say it out loud! Say it with me. NO! If it doesn't work on the first try, say it out loud again. Usually, by the third time I've said NO!, the food fixation goes away. I don't really know why it works — don't care. It works.

Another tip is one that was given to me by a nurse who helped me in my recovery following my accident. She liked to analyze the little food predators by using the HATTS method. HATTS stands for Hungry, Angry, Thirsty, Tired, Stressed. At the moment the gnawing need to have a snack creeps up on you, ask yourself whether you are hungry, angry, thirsty, tired, or stressed. If you're one or more of those things at that moment, attempt to relieve the condition by a more appropriate method than eating, and the food yearning should go away. If it doesn't, start yelling, "NO! NO! NO! NO!" at the top of your lungs, and then run for about a block. That may not help either, but it at least got you a block away from the food!

Now running from food is not what you want to be doing very often. You need to learn to control the food, and to control your actual "need" for food. The only real control food should have over you is the fact that it keeps you alive, keeps your weight moving down, and keeps your hair in your head.

But the brain is a funny and complex thing, and it likes to play horrible tricks on us. You will grapple for a long time with getting your eyes and brain to communicate with your pouch/stomach as to the proper amount of food it will hold. Your "eyes being too big for your stomach" will be something that is hard to equalize.

In the beginning you will not want any food. Then you'll only want a little food, which isn't enough. Then when you can really eat food, and you're getting the hang of what foods work, you get a bit complacent, and you start eating like a normal person again. Not eating like you used to, just eating like a normal person.

You're not a normal person though. You're plumbed differently. You need to eat less than normal people. You will often just take too much food, and figure out you can't eat it. Case in point: the buffet story in Chapter Nine. Karen and I still take too much food on occasion. Inevitably one asks the other, "Exactly what *were* you thinking when you did that?" Then, if at all possible, we feed the rest to my husband Matt. (Why feed the garbage-god when you can feed the human garbage disposal?)

Anyway, you deal with it and move on. But here's a tip that might help: when I am eating at home (and not eating plastic food), I have learned to eat my food on a salad plate rather than a dinner plate. I can't fill it up as much, and it still looks full.

Now I know many of you have tried this trick in the past, but it didn't work then because you still had room in your stomach. You simply went back and filled up the salad plate again (and maybe again). But it works now because of the limited amount of space in your pouch/stomach.

The problem in my house became that as soon as I started using the salad plates all the time, so did my husband for some stupid reason! What the heck?! Did I start a new fad or something? So I went out and bought a box of eight cheap, clear glass salad plates, and that kind of kept the supply healthy in between running the dishwasher and Matt's four PB&J sandwiches per day.

If you have lapses in putting the proper amount of food on your plate, and you have no human garbage disposal spouse, or growing child to feed it to, just stick it in a container and call it leftovers. At least it will be easy pickin's for another day's protein safari.

Living a life on the protein safari is simply a matter of trial, error, and environmental adaptation. It's like moving to a big city, or a new country: you simply have to live there a while, grumble a bit about how different things are, and then figure out how to make it work for you in order to get you what you need, and where you need to go. Adjust.

So, in conclusion, the protein safari, like everything else in your life after weight loss surgery, it has an annoyance and an amusement factor. The trick is making the amusement factor outweigh the annoyance factor. Any time you think the annoyance factor is winning, sit down and review your personal list of little victories. That will put it all in perspective for you, and prepare you for another fun-filled day of tracking big-game on the safari.

Happy hunting!

Chapter Thirteen

— THE JUNK DRAWER —

Julie M. Janeway
Karen J. Sparks

This chapter is the book's junk drawer. Everybody has a junk drawer, right? It's the place where you put the stuff that doesn't really have any other place to live. Shoelaces, ticket stubs, odd batteries, tape, rubber bands, your old glasses, loose change, etc., are the kinds of things you find in the junk drawer. Most of them are useful for you or someone else, but they are all unrelated items residing in one space.

So, that's what we put in this chapter: all the things that had no other place to go, are useful to you or someone else, and are basically unrelated to each other. They're now all sharing one space, so if this chapter seems a bit messy and disconnected, that's what it was designed to be. Please bear with us as we've basically just tossed in all this information that has no other home. It will just sit here until you need it, minding it's own business. But, when you're looking for it later, hopefully you'll remember to check the junk drawer first.

Hidden Costs Related to Weight Loss

Where to start? Well maybe from the bottom up? Let's start with shoes. When you lose a tremendous amount of weight, as you should with bariatric surgery, your feet get smaller. So, you may find that you move from wide width shoes to regular width shoes. You will just wake up one day, and when you put your shoes on, you'll walk right out of them because they're too big.

Now that's a bit of a tick-off when they are your favorite shoes! But this is kind of the cost of doing business: you will have to start replacing your shoes. But wait, there's more! Not only may your feet shrink from wide width to regular width, but the length of your feet may actually change as well! No, really!

I've worn a size 10 medium shoe all my life — since I was in fifth grade. I rarely had to wear wide shoes, but I always needed a 10 for the length. By the time I lost about 100 pounds, I noticed that all of my size 10 shoes were starting to just sort of flop around on my feet. It wasn't that they were too wide, it was that they were too long, and I was walking out of them.

Now I wear a size 9 or 9½ shoe. Go figure! I've had to begin replacing my shoes because the 10s just won't stay on. That was an expense I hadn't counted on. Few people do.

And here's another one you might not see coming: socks and hosiery. You shrink out of all that too. Socks maybe only once or twice, but with hosiery you'll shrink down several sizes, so don't buy in bulk, because you'll either shrink through and not wear them, or you'll be stuck wearing hose with baggy "elephant" ankles. Don't waste the money. Buy as you go.

This next one is really more for the women reading this than the men because it deals with underwear. We know it to be an undisputed fact that men will not buy new underwear no matter what the conditions or circumstances. Men will tie their underwear on with a shoelace, or tape it on with duct tape before they'll buy new underwear.

Women, however, will need to buy new undies at least two or three times during the weight loss period. Now the undies you can handle unless you're addicted to expensive undies from the "lady with the secret" store, but the real kicker is replacing your bras. That gets expensive. You don't realize how that adds up until you've replaced them for the third or more time. Again, it's also a real drag because we always have our favorite bra, the one that doesn't pinch, bind, or pull, and you will hate having to say goodbye to it. Not only does it not pinch, bind, or pull, it doesn't lift, shape, or separate anymore either. Lets hope it has a twin in a smaller size.

Related to underwear are bathing suits. Nobody really thinks about this one, unless you live in a climate in which you can wear a bathing suit all year 'round. In Michigan, we only have summer for about ten minutes each year (somewhere in July), so we don't spend much time in bathing suits. So when you have one on in July, and then you don't have it on again until next July, and you've lost 150 pounds over the year, the bathing suit has to be replaced.

If you live in a climate that is conducive to year 'round bathing suit wearing, then you'll probably have to replace this item more than once as you shrink. You may have more sunshine and warm weather year 'round, but we can spend less money on replacing bathing suits, so there!

When you get out of the pool in your bathing suit, or you get out of the shower, you put on your…what? ROBE. That's right. Yes, you'll have to replace your robe too. When you are actually wrapping it around and it's meeting in the back, no belt in the world is going to hold it in place. Your favorite, comfy, squishy, warm robe will have to go in the pile of too big garments with all your other favorite things. Again, this tidbit is only for women, as we know men will not buy a new robe, EVER, assuming they own one in the first place.

If you've had your swim, and you've had your shower, maybe now you'd like to put on your jammies and go to bed. Oh…but wait…they're too big too. So now you'll have to replace your pajamas. The good news ladies, is that you can make your nightgowns last quite a while, but at some point they'll get so big you'll actually squirm out of the neck of them during the night. Also, when the sleepwear gets really big, the significant other isn't finding it quite so attractive and alluring, if you know what I mean.

Now this little problem is no problem at all if you sleep in the buff, but you'll have to buy at least one sleepwear item to keep in your stash in case you're ever in a hotel and it catches on fire. Everyone (men too), needs to own a set of "hotel fire" jammies. Speaking of hotel fires, when you see them on T.V., there's always people who didn't bring their hotel fire jammies, and have to stand around with their coat on (or someone else's coat on), so they don't have to hide behind a bush while the fire is being put out. That brings us to the next thing that costs money: coats.

Coats have to be replaced as well. I had a most favorite coat, that I affectionately called my "teddy" coat. It was a suede coat in the shearling style, but it was completely lined (pockets too) in the softest fake fur you've ever felt. It's the kind of fur they use to make teddy bears for newborn babies. I bought it two weeks before my surgery, because I didn't know I'd be having surgery that soon. If I'd known I'd have to give it up so soon after adopting it, I would have saved myself the grief and sorrow.

I just adored that coat. It was the warmest, most cuddly coat I'd ever owned, even though it was a size 4x. I had my surgery on October 29, 2003, and by March of 2004, I could wrap the coat around me and tuck each side underneath the opposite arm. I absolutely did not want to give up my teddy coat. I searched and searched, and to this day have not been able to find another one exactly like it. Finally, in April of 2004, as the ice was beginning to melt and a hint of spring was in the air, I found the courage to part with my beloved teddy coat.

Last fall, however, I had to begin the hunt for a new teddy coat. On top of the fact that I just needed a teddy coat because I missed it, I'd lost a lot of weight and now had the thermostat issue we wrote about in Chapter Four. I'm always cold, so I needed a really warm coat. I hunted, and hunted, but no teddy coat. Oh sure, many masqueraded as teddy coats (only partial teddy fur lining), and there were plenty of teddy coat wannabes, but alas, no teddy coat for Julie.

Then one day, there it was. Not my teddy coat, but a close relative. My teddy coat was tan, and this coat was black. I approached with cautious optimism, not knowing if I could handle another disappointment. I'd searched so long, so hard. I didn't dare hope that this could be the teddy coat I'd devoted my life to finding.

Reaching out, I touched the fur lining expecting to feel the scrape of cheap, imitation teddy fur. But to my surprise, I found the feel of the teddy fur I remembered. Could it be that this was merely a darker version of my cherished teddy coat? Indeed, it was! Oh, joy! My teddy coat had been found, and it was not a size 4x, but simply a misses size large.

Finding my teddy coat meant I would be warm, and it gave me high hopes of surviving the winter after all. My husband was relieved to know that I wouldn't freeze to death in the driveway before reaching my car. All was again right with the world.

But what of my first teddy coat, you ask? What was its fate? Well, at first it was reluctantly boxed up for sale, but I couldn't bear to part with it, and I felt so guilty putting it away in that cold, lonely box. So, I staged a daring rescue while my husband was away, and now it fulfills a new role in my life: lap blanket. Yes, once again my teddy coat has found purpose and contentment, and I have enjoyed its warm and soft embrace. Together we watch television, read books, and cuddle with the cats. My original teddy coat and I have been reunited, and today my teddy coats and I are living happily ever after.

Replacing your coat is not the end of the line, however. Did it occur to you that your head shrinks too? Yep. It shrinks. If you have nothing in your wardrobe but adjustable baseball caps, then you're probably going to luck out on this one. If, however, you like fitted caps, or have other hats in your accessory wardrobe, you will likely find that they'll end up too big, and they'll have to be replaced.

It doesn't stop with hats though. Let's examine other members of the accessory wardrobe family, shall we? Jewelry also becomes obsolete. Of course we're not suggesting that you ditch your wedding rings, toss your grandmother's locket, or dump the bracelet you received as an anniversary present. What we are telling you is that you may find that your jewelry is now out of scale to your new size. I know that because I was always a big person, and I always wore quite big jewelry so it looked like it "fit." By the time I lost about 80 to 90 pounds, I found that my jewelry was really just too big, and was overpowering both my outfits and me.

The obvious solution is to run right out and buy all new fine jewelry, right?! After all, diamonds go with everything you know.... But when you wake up from that dream, you figure out that you simply need to begin working on replacing things one piece at a time. Costume jewelry is good, but if you can afford it, buy yourself a nice piece of "real" jewelry as a reward every once in a while, because you deserve it.

Another tip from "Moi," the jewelry queen herself, is instead of rushing out and having your rings resized to your newly slim fingers, refrain from resizing for awhile. First of all, your fingers shrink quite a bit. I lost three rings sizes, so if I had my rings resized every time I shrank a ring size, it would have cost me, on average, about ten dollars per sizing, per ring. That really adds up if you're a jewelry maven like me! I would have had to mortgage my house to pay for my ring resizing!

What I did instead, was to go to a pawnshop that sells jewelry, and look for very thin, plain gold bands. I found ones that fit my new finger size, and now wear them in front of my other rings to hold them on. You really can't see them, they hold your rings on quite well, they can be used over and over again with different rings, and they cost about $6 per band (10k gold). It's much cheaper than paying for repeated ring resizing, and you don't lose all the gold that is taken out of your rings!

So I've given you a good little tip on jewelry resizing, but I don't really have any good tips on inexpensively replacing your glasses. Your glasses may get too big for your slimmed down face, and that means your sunglasses as well. Sunglasses, if they aren't prescription, aren't too hard to replace. Heck, even the dollar stores carry sunglasses! But prescription glasses are another story, especially if you don't have optical coverage. We suggest keeping a close eye (no pun intended) on the specials offered at various optical centers, especially Sears® and D.O.C. (Detroit Optometric Center), as it runs some pretty amazing sales throughout the year.

And…speaking of things that go on your face, don't forget the expense that comes with buying new make-up for the ladies, and skin care products for both men and women. Once you begin to shrink, your face will change shape, and you may begin to see some lines where there were none before. You may also begin to see some droopy skin, or some hanging skin under your chin. This may be helped without the aid of plastic surgery, or Botox® injections simply by purchasing a quality moisturizer with sunscreen, and a skin firming product containing collagen, elastin, and/or Q10.

Many such products exist, but we suggest not heading for the cheapest thing on the market. Your looks are important to your self-esteem (men too), and you should buy a product that will give you the best benefit, not just one that will be easy on your wallet.

Don't buy cheap moisturizers either. We can't overemphasize the need to keep your skin moisturized from the outside, and hydrated from the inside. The drier your skin is, the more it will wrinkle, bag, and sag. Moist, firm skin looks younger and healthier. Even if you have oily skin, there are appropriate moisturizing products out there for you. Men, don't ignore me here! You need moisture too. Drink your water, and slap some moisturizer on your face and body. Your shrinking skin will thank you.

Not only does your skin need to be cared for while you shrink, but your hair does as well. We've already talked about the hair loss issue in Chapter Six, and we've clued you in to the fact that you should take the opportunity to update your look, whether or not you have hair loss issues. Many of us thought that we needed more hair to balance out our heads with our big bodies. I always referred to people with small heads and large bodies as illustrating the "peanut on a pumpkin" effect. Men do this too by growing their hair long, or wearing an outdated style that's just plain out of shape.

As you shrink, however, the proportion between your head and your body changes, and you may find that you don't need all that hair. We suggest going to any clothing store, and standing at least fifteen feet from a full-length mirror. This will let you appraise yourself as a whole person, rather than focusing simply on the bad or the good parts. Then look at the proportions of your hair to your head, and your head to your body. Take a friend who'll be brutally honest with you, and listen to what he or she has to say. Then make an appointment with a good stylist, cut that hair a bit, and update your look.

When you're done, don't sit in the chair three feet from the mirror. Get up and stand 15 feet away and honestly evaluate how your new cut looks in relation to your face, and in relation to the proportions of your body. Maybe it's the first cut, and maybe it won't be the last. Re-evaluate periodically as you shrink. In any event, you're bound to feel much lighter and incredibly better about yourself, if not a little more broke.

And… with the concept of being broke, comes the biggest offender of them all: replacing your general wardrobe. One of the best things that happens to you when you lose weight is that you shrink and therefore move into smaller size clothing. One of the worst things that happens to you when you lose weight is that you shrink and therefore move into smaller size clothing.

Most people when they lose weight only lose one or two sizes, and that means many things can be altered down. When weight loss surgery patients lose weight they generally lose a minimum of four sizes. I lost seven sizes going from a 28 to a 14. Karen lost ten sizes going from 34 to a 14. The average garment can only be altered a maximum of two sizes. I'll wait while you do the math.

Obviously, when you repeatedly shrink right through every thing you own, it's not realistic to keep replacing it over and over again. But it's also not realistic to keep wearing clothes that are literally hanging off you either. So what do you do? Well here are a few tips.

First, one of the obvious benefits of having surgery done through a multi-disciplinary practice is that they provide support groups. Aside from the intended purpose of the support groups, they allow you to meet other people who are approximately your size, and who have gone through the surgery before you or after you. What this facilitates is finding people with whom to "buddy-up" on a clothing co-op. As one shrinks out of something, another can shrink into it.

You don't spend very long in any one size, so the clothing certainly doesn't take a beating. In fact, as we've stated before, many of the items will pass to new owners without even having had the tags removed. It helps tremendously to know that clothing exists to get you to work and other events, and that you don't have to sell a kidney in order to pay for your clothing replacement needs.

As Karen and I went through this process, we buddied-up on almost everything. She knew that when I shrunk out of something, it was only a matter of weeks before she knew she'd shrink into it. (Remember her surgery was six weeks behind mine.) In fact, at one point Karen realized that I was buying all the replacement clothes for myself, while she was simply shrinking into mine. I couldn't find anyone to be on the giving end so I could be on the receiving end, as no other patients we met had jobs that required them to dress as formally for their jobs as we did. So, Karen started buying me some clothes because she knew that it was only a matter of time before they came to her, many having never been worn. At least that way we split the cost.

Now we didn't always have just one of any particular item waiting to go through the system. Occasionally we found something both of us wanted at the same time. Generally that desire was made stronger by the fact that it was on serious sale at the time as well. Case in point: the periwinkle blazer.

The first spring after our surgeries we both found a beautiful periwinkle blazer on sale for $29.99. We simply both had to have one as we both look great in that color (doesn't everybody though…?) So we both bought a blazer, and Karen knew that when I shrunk out of mine, I would be out of luck, and she'd be up one new blazer.

Well that time came within a few weeks, and I had to say goodbye to my new blazer. It wasn't quite as sad a parting as I'd had with my teddy coat, because I could visit it every once in a while. My blazer left me and moved in with Karen. Karen shrunk into that blazer and she enjoyed wearing it. I, however, was periwinkle blazer-less, and feeling a little moody about it.

So one day, on another of our famous "important woman business" shopping trips, I found another periwinkle blazer, but it was now on sale for $19.99. What luck! I immediately bought it knowing full well that Karen would be able to continue wearing periwinkle blazers far longer than I, and soon she would own this one too.

I stayed in that blazer for a little longer than the first, but eventually it joined its predecessor at Karen's house. Again I went into mourning for my blazer. A few weeks later, Karen had been out of town for a meeting and found yet another periwinkle blazer in a smaller size, and this time it was on clearance for $12.99! She bought it for me, and I was happy for the remainder of the summer. But that happiness was again shortlived. It seemed like only minutes before that blazer was moving out to join its kin at Karen's house. It seemed Karen was destined to remain perfectly clad in periwinkle.

I never saw another periwinkle blazer like that one again, but Karen ultimately ended up with full legal custody of four periwinkle blazers in descending sizes; none of which either one of us can wear anymore or have tailored down. We've since resolved not to engage in that type of behavior again. We've set the maximum legal limit for exact copies of clothing at two. Any more than that is just plain crazy.

In order not to appear crazy, and not to keep spending a ton of money on replacement clothes, here are a few more tips on how to get through this dilemma. First, when buying clothes, buy only on sale, or better yet "clearance," unless it's for a special occasion. Don't buy expensive clothes, or investment pieces until you're almost done, or completely done shrinking. You'll just have to say goodbye to more expensive clothing, and more money lost. Also, don't discount shopping at garage sales, resale stores, and consignment shops. Many good bargains are there for the taking.

Second, buy only separate pieces (not suits or matching outfits) and get very good at mixing and matching pieces. If you buy one piece of clothing to match only with another in order to make a specific outfit, you'll be bored, and your wardrobe will be severely limited. Also, if you shrink out of half of the outfit (and you will as parts of you will shrink at different rates than others), what will you do with the other half? Make sure to buy solid color, or minimal print pieces so that you can mix and match for maximum usage.

Third, when buying clothing, make sure that you buy clothes that have a lot of seams. Jackets should have back seams, and preferably princess seaming in the front and back. If you don't know what princess seaming is, ask a salesperson at a store. Remember that pieces can only be altered a maximum of two sizes. The more seams, and/or darts a piece has, the easier it is to have it altered if you really want to get maximum wear-time out of it.

Also, take the time to find a good tailor who charges reasonable rates. Many good tailors are out there, but some of them charge exorbitant rates. You could replace the item two or three times for what they want to cut it down one size. Do your shopping, and ask around. People with tailoring shops are not usually your best bet. Tailors or dressmakers who work from their homes generally charge less expensive rates.

Tailors generally can take care of more than one of the problems that arise, however, and that is as your clothes get bigger, they also get longer. If a skirt begins to get bigger, it gets longer too, so have the dressmaker take the skirt in, and shorten it at the same time.

Also, ladies you'll notice that as you begin to hit about size 18 or 16, many of the plus size clothes seem very long, especially blazers, t-shirts, and sweaters. If you think I'm kidding, put your clothes on and stand fifteen feet from a full-length mirror.

Look at the proportions of your clothes. Now get your trusty friend (the one who'll be brutally honest), to pin up the hem of the skirt, or the bottom of the jacket or shirt a few inches. Get the sleeve lengths where they should be (approximately ½-¾ of an inch above the thumb knuckle where it connects to the hand). Now look at the proportions on your body. You probably look smaller and taller. Clothes that are too long in proportion simply make you look heavier, and dowdier.

Another way to examine this is to have a friend take digital photos of you. This also helps with wrapping your head around what size you really are, and what you really look like at a particular point in time. The reason this works is because mirrors lie, and our minds lie. If you stand less than six feet from a mirror, your mind will play tricks on you. Some days you'll think you look like a million bucks, and other days you'll think you look like you haven't lost a pound.

Similarly, the mind has a set configuration for recognizing itself, and it will often conform the images being viewed to that configuration. This is one of the basic reasons people look in the mirror and can't see the drastic changes (good or bad) that others see.

People who were thin for most of their lives, can't really see how much weight they've put on until they see a picture of themselves because it's not actual size, like it is in a mirror. In the same vein, those who've been heavy all their lives, have the similar difficulties in adjusting their view of themselves as thinner people. It's hard to adjust this "gestalt." Pictures really help us figure out what image to have of ourselves now.

So you may be able to grasp the fact that you've lost weight, but don't get hung up on the numbers printed on the tag on your clothes. You must realize that women's clothes are not like men's. Men's clothes are generally based on actual measurements (17 inch neck, 34 inch waist, 32 inch inseam).

Women's clothing sizes are based on the "fit model" used to create the original patterns. In regular misses sizes, the female model used to fit the original pattern is generally one of those stick figures that walks down the runway in New York. The original pattern is generally a size six, and will be dependent on that model's particular body shape, and the cut of the garment.

The manufacturers then usually take the pattern and simply size it up proportionately for each size after size six. So, it's sort of like tracing one inch all the way around it to get the next size, and then tracing one inch all the way around that to get the following size, etc., etc.

Plus sizes generally work the same way except that they normally use a plus size model who is a size 12 or 14, and again the fit is dependent on how the model is proportioned. That's why some pants are bigger in the body and slimmer in the legs, and others are cut more fully through the hips and thighs. It depends on where the "fit model" carried her weight, and the cut of the garment.

If the "fit model" was in between a 12 and a 14, maybe the manufacturer just picked a number, we'll call it a 14, and then went up from there. That's why it may fit smaller than other size 14 clothes by other makers. If the manufacturer cut the garment and called it a 12, however, the garment will fit bigger than garments marked the same size. So what's the point of all this trivia? To let you know that you must shop in a range of three sizes. I can wear anything from a misses size 14 to an 18, or a size 14w to a 16w, and on occasion an 18w if it really fits small.

I don't flip out any more about what the tag says. I go for fit and comfort (and more importantly sale price), more so than what size it says on the tag. Our clothes aren't standardized like men's because they aren't based on actual inch measurements. So stop beating yourself up about what the tag says. The general size that you "are" at any given moment is where you average out in clothes.

I average out at a misses size 14 on the top, and a women's size 14 or a regular 16 on the bottom. As long as I'm not consistently moving up in clothing sizes, I'm okay. We all want to be able to shrink into the next smaller size, but don't get stuck on that. It is okay though to buy something (especially if it's on clearance) that is a bit too small, and hang it in your closet as "goal" clothing. You'll shrink into it soon enough.

In conclusion, I will tell you that losing a large amount of weight is very expensive. I will also tell you, however, that your food budget goes down considerably, and you won't be spending that $50 to $60 a week you were spending in the drive-thru or at restaurants. You won't be getting richer, but if you stop and look at it, you will have a little more money left over to help you with some of these expenses. Be creative, be frugal, and be happy you've lost the weight and are healthier, no matter what it might cost or how inconvenient it might be.

Pre-Op Emotional Issues

Well, we've told you about many of the other types of emotional issues you may experience if you have weight loss surgery, but we haven't really discussed the emotional upheaval you may experience during the 24 to 48 hours beforehand. During this time you begin to really grapple with the fact that you're finally going to give up some control of your eating, your weight, and your related medical conditions to other people. You may have thought you were okay with that, but in those hours before surgery it really begins to sink in that you're going to have to let these people help you, you're going to have to let them in and pay attention to what they say, and that this is a one way ride.

You also really begin to deal with the fact that you may finally be getting what you've always wanted: permanent relief from the nastiness that comes with being overweight. You will likely start to examine that in *ad nauseum* detail, mulling over whether this is really what you want or not. You think you've given it significant consideration thus far? You haven't even begun the mulling process yet until you hit those last hours before the O.R.

The last hours are when it becomes overwhelmingly real. Many patients begin to face the possibility, albeit a statistically insignificant possibility, that they could die from surgery. You know it is a possibility, and you also know that it's a remote possibility, but still it hits you squarely between the eyes and throws you for a loop.

The fear of the pain begins to creep in, and you remind yourself over and over again that there's medication for that. You begin to concentrate on the fact that your anatomy is going to be changed pretty much irreversibly, and you're no longer going to be in the condition your Maker made you. You may just begin to fear the details of everything.

The fear of change really moves in and sets up housekeeping as well. You start to think about all the things that may become different, and strangely you don't necessarily see them as being positive anymore. You may find yourself clinging to the familiar because it's a known quantity. When the fear sets in you must keep reminding yourself, and have others remind you as well, "You can do anything afraid, that you can do unafraid." If that doesn't work, try "Always, always, always, always, always do what you are afraid to do." This is also a time to find your faith, whatever it may be, and hold on to that. It will help with the fear and emotional overload now and down the road, more than you know.

For some people the emotions are all over the map; happiness, sadness, fear, panic. For others it is manifested in sheer elation. This has never been more apparent to me than when I had my surgery and I was in the holding room right outside the O.R. In that room there are about twelve beds with people waiting to go in for various types of surgeries. It doesn't matter what type of surgery you're having, you may still go through this type of fear, analysis, emotional turmoil, and second-guessing.

When I was waiting to be brought to the O.R., I noticed other people who were waiting to have weight loss surgery done by Dr. Baker's partners. They appeared to be everything from happy and excited, to crying and scared, and one was almost morose. Personally, I was freaking out because despite the number of other surgeries I'd had in the previous two and a half years, I began to have flashbacks to my accident and the first night they took me into surgery. I wasn't prepared for that. I thought I had the fear of surgery licked. I thought I had it under control and it was a no-brainer. I was wrong.

I guess it kicked in for me because deep down I knew this surgery was going to be as life altering as the first one after my accident. That one determined whether I lived or died, walked or didn't walk. This one also determined, in a way, whether I really "lived" or not. I didn't expect the terror, the uncontrolled panic and hysteria, and the feeling that I wanted to leave as fast as I could, and didn't even care where I went. I wasn't prepared for any of that, and that scared me even more.

Intellectually, I knew that this surgery was a good thing that it was the right thing, but emotions are pretty unpredictable little monsters, and they gave me a great big "gotcha." Others in the room were very confused, and kept asking nurses what kind of surgery I was having done. Other weight loss surgery patients, especially the ones that were happy and excited, were a bit perplexed, and I fear I kind of made them second guess their own happiness and commitment to going forward. Oooops! Sorry.

But as we keep telling you, each person is radically different from the next. We can't predict for you how you'll react, just know that you will and it's okay to do so. Karen, for example, was also a basket case. She was hit by a wave of emotion she and her family weren't prepared for either. She couldn't stop crying, she was terrified of the change coming in her life, and she was overwhelmed by the fear of the unknown.

Karen had such a death grip on her mom and me that I still have the scars on my fingers where she was squeezing my hand, and the diamonds on my wedding band cut my fingers open. I did finally manage to wrangle myself free and seek some medical attention for that (and an x-ray…), but I still feel bad about leaving her poor little mom to fend for herself. Sorry about that Mrs. Sparks.

Dr. Baker and his Physician Assistants, Matt and Randy, were entirely supportive and understanding, and helped both Karen and me during those last moments before going into surgery. They made sure that we got a little something to help calm us down before we went in. It was a good thing too, as after I got Karen to release the Vulcan Death Grip on my hand, she clamped onto the bed rail, and would have been responsible for replacing an expensive piece of medical equipment had she not started to relax just as the metal was about to snap!

Just as with my experience, there were several others waiting to go to surgery when Karen was in the pre-op holding area. This one particular woman was so excited she could hardly contain herself, and she just couldn't understand why Karen was upset and scared. She kept trying to talk to Karen and ask her questions. Karen was torn between telling this woman to just shut-up and leave her alone, and hiding under the covers. Fortunately they have those curtains you can draw around the bed as I feared it would have been the former rather than the latter, and it wouldn't have been any too polite or quiet.

So to draw this section to a close, we just want you to know that whatever range of emotions you feel, and whatever decides to jump up and down on you in those last hours before surgery, know that it is perfectly normal, and all will work out the way it is supposed to work out. Keep supportive, loving people close to you, let your medical team know exactly what you're feeling and let them help you, and take pity on those who offer to hold your hand. We're only here to help; paralysis and scarring isn't part of the bargain.

Surgical and Physical Issues

We're moving from pre-op to post-op now. The first thing we want to emphasize is that you must do what they ask you to do from the moment you wake up from surgery. They will ask you to get out of bed and walk around sometime within twelve hours after surgery. No, you will not want to get up and walk, but you have to anyway. It's for your own good.

Walking helps to get the blood flowing again, and prevents blood clots from forming. Walking also gets you breathing, helps to move the anesthetic out of your lungs and system, and helps to re-inflate your lungs so you won't have a pulmonary collapse. Walking is good, even if it doesn't feel good.

The next important piece of advice we can give you is to accurately and calmly assess your pain level (on a scale of 1 to 10, with 10 being the worst pain you've ever felt in your life), and report it to your nurse. Don't try and be a big brave soldier. You must break the pain cycle, and keep it broken. If they give you one of those little jeopardy buttons (PCA – patient controlled analgesic device) for the pain, then use it. You can't overdose on it. It's regulated, and you can press the thing all you want, but it will only give you a measured dose at set time intervals. So if it is set for every ten minutes, you can push the button like there's no tomorrow, and it will only give you the correct dosage every ten minutes.

Breaking the pain cycle is important. If you doze off, and you will, press it as soon as you wake up. You'll fall asleep and you'll think you've been asleep for hours, but you may find it's only been eight minutes. Press the button anyway. It can't hurt, but it can help.

If you don't have a PCA, make sure to tell the nurse when you're becoming painful again. Don't try and tough it out. There's no point to that, unless you have some weird affinity for pain and suffering. If that's the case, you have bigger problems than being overweight. Just take the medication. You are not receiving enough to become addicted.

Dr. Baker says that even if you've had problems with pain medication addiction in the past, make sure that your doctor is aware of the issue, and it will be handled in an appropriate manner. Just because you've had a problem with addiction does not mean that you have to suffer through the pain with no help. Trust your medical team to know what to do to help you.

Also, when you go home, your doctor will most likely send you with some form of pain medication, probably in liquid form (for which you will be grateful). Follow the instructions and take the pain medication. Remember that we told you the pain is worst on days two through five. Be aware, however, that medication tends to get into the bloodstream pretty fast after gastric bypass surgery, not unlike alcohol. So from the perspective of pain relief it works quite fast, but also know that other medications may kick in quite quickly too. Whether or not that is an issue is something you should discuss with your physician before surgery.

After surgery, the medical staff may also want you to breathe into the spirometer (the little device that you breathe in to make the balls move up and down). Although it may seem stupid, and it may seem hard to do, or cause some pain in your diaphragm, please don't ignore this little treatment. You don't have to do it forever, just for a couple of days. Take pity on your little lungs, and your whole body for that matter, and just be compliant. It's really quite necessary, and it is not designed just to annoy you, or just for the sake of being a pain in the neck. Waking you up to tell you to go to sleep, now that is designed to annoy you, and is just for the sake of being a pain in the neck!!!

So the moral of this story is: Do as you are told. Gee, just like mom said all those years ago. Again, they're not doing it for the good of their health, they're doing it for the good of yours. More wise words from my sister Cheryl: "They are not the enemy."

Julie and Karen's Personal Theories About Stuff

Let me just say right off that this is a totally unscientific, untested, unfounded, unresearched portion of the book. These are 100% our personal observations, and they have no scientific merit whatsoever. That being said, we will also say that they have proven to work over and over again, so we do claim some form of validity and reliability in our totally non-scientific experiments.

The first theory has developed from an experiment I have been running for about the last thirty years of my life. Karen is new to the experiment, but she can report that she has been able to reproduce my results on a consistent basis. This theory is called the Skinny Mirror Theory.

For the last 30 or so years I have been testing just about any mirror I encounter to determine whether the mirror reflects an accurate image of me, or whether it reflects a slightly modified, somewhat "fun house" version of what I look like by making me appear taller and slimmer than I really am while not completely distorting the image.

Many such mirrors exist, and they should be noted as to their locations across the country. I've noticed that mid-priced to expensive clothing stores tend to invest in the placement of skinny mirrors throughout their facilities. I believe they understand the psychology behind the use of skinny mirrors in that customers tend to buy just about anything that makes them look thinner, no matter how hideous it may in fact be. Less expensive stores don't seem to care, they just hope you'll buy anything.

The danger in skinny mirrors is exactly as I've just stated: you may be prone to buying anything that makes you look thinner, no matter how hideous it might be. So although having a skinny mirror in your home is a wonderful, life-affirming thing, be mindful that the skinny mirrors in stores can have an hallucinogenic effect that may inhibit your judgment and impulse control.

To prevent skinny mirrors from inappropriately affecting your buying habits, be sure to stand at least fifteen feet from all full length mirrors in stores when evaluating a potential clothing purchase. This tends to negate the "overthinning" effect of the skinny mirror, and the attendant cascade of whatever brain chemicals are involved in the rabid buying behavior that goes on after that.

Skinny mirrors, however, make wonderful home companions. Once appropriate clothing has been purchased (by that we mean it is not hideous and has not been purchased while under the influence of a skinny mirror), the home skinny mirror will become a trusted friend that sends you on your way every day with a positive attitude and a spring in your step.

As a word of caution, "fat mirrors" also exist, and these are to be avoided at all costs. In the event a home skinny mirror cannot be located and procured, a regular accurate mirror will serve in its place until an appropriate replacement can be found. Under no circumstances should a fat mirror ever reside in your home whether by purchase or by gift. Fat mirrors are evil and should be destroyed on sight.

The next theory we've developed is called the Ketchup Theory. The Ketchup Theory is a fairly new theory for us, and like the rest of the theories that follow, were developed solely post-surgery. Although it involves ketchup, don't discount it off the bat if you are not a ketchup lover. It also involves other substances made with tomatoes, but the term "Ketchup, Tomato Soup, Tomato Sauce, Tomatoes, Salsa, Pizza Sauce Theory," was just a bit too long and unwieldy.

The Ketchup Theory deals with the effect that comes from eating foods accompanied by tomato-based products. We find, and we've asked others too, that foods tend to sit better and not fight back as much, if they are accompanied by a tomato-based product. As we said, there's no scientific proof for this, but we prefer to believe that it is because of the acid in the tomatoes.

As the new little pouch has virtually no acid makers in it at all (they're all in the remainder of the stomach), we think that the acid helps with breaking down the food a bit before it reaches the true stomach acid down in the small bowel. There may be no truth to this at all, but all we know is that whenever we eat food with a bit of ketchup (including the occasional french fry or two), the food sits better.

I can eat a few french fries if I dip them in ketchup. If I eat more than two french fries without ketchup, they just don't sit well and I'm quite uncomfortable for a while. Now, the Ketchup Theory is not professing to allow you to eat a whole order of french fries. It will not do that for you, and you shouldn't be doing that anyway. If you do, you probably deserve the auto eject experience you're going to have.

What it does seem to do is allow you to eat a few fries so you feel like a regular person, without sending you into cramps or auto eject. Similarly, a bit of low-fat or fat-free spaghetti sauce on chicken gives it a nice flavor and helps it go down quite well. A cup of tomato soup (with actual tomatoes), and a half of a wrap sandwich seems to work out quite well also. So don't run out and cover everything in the world in ketchup or tomato sauces. Remember that they have calories and other ingredients too, not the least of which is often a high sugar content. If you're allergic to food acids like I am, then be careful in your consumption, and keep some anti-histamines handy.

The next theory is somewhat related to the Ketchup Theory, and is called the "Greasing the Skids Theory." By "greasing the skids" we mean making sure that you've had something to drink (preferably water) at least ten to fifteen minutes before you eat, and if you haven't, then grease the skids by adding in some form of light liquid as part of the meal itself. I'll explain.

As Carrie and Dr. Baker told you, you should drink before meals, and then about an hour after meals. The drinking before meals helps to control the need to tear into your food. But we've also found that if you don't have much liquid in the system, things might just get stuck in the pipes.

If I get up in the morning and eat something without having had at least a half a bottle of water first, it just gets stuck, and then it hurts. I hate starting my day that way. Then I had the brilliant idea of just starting the day by eating a yogurt. After all, it is liquid, right? That didn't work well either. I made myself quite ill. I guess it's more solid than liquid or something.

From our experiences, it works best if you just drink some water and let it sit a couple of minutes before you eat. "But what if I can't drink ten to fifteen minutes before I eat? What if I'm not in a position to do that?" you ask. Well then the second half of the theory comes into play. We suggest, and we're not giving you a license to go crazy here, that you might have a bit of gravy on the side to dip meat into, or a small cup of soup with the meal, not before.

Maybe a little mustard or salsa (there's that Ketchup Theory again) could be put to use to make meat or other foods a bit more "wet." Do not, however, drown anything in sauces or condiments. Dipping is okay, drowning in it is not. You're just "greasing" the skids a little, not submerging them in liquid.

And speaking of liquid, that brings us to our final theory, the "Tea Theory." The Tea Theory is very similar in nature to the Ketchup Theory in that it involves our suppositions regarding the tannic acid in tea. Now we're referring to tea as being either iced or hot, but not containing lemon. We have found, and almost every single person we've talked to has had the same response, that citric acid tends to be too strong and isn't tolerated well after weight loss surgery. Citric acid is the type of acid found in citrus fruits like lemons, oranges, limes, and grapefruits.

Tea contains tannic acid, however, which appears to be somewhat on the strength of the acid in tomato-based products, and it seems to do the same thing. The difference is that you ingest it about an hour after eating, not while eating. The caution that comes with this theory, is to refrain from drinking it while eating, and from drinking too much of it. Not only does it contain caffeine, but if consumed in large quantities, it does contain a significant amount of acid that can adversely affect your bones. Also, it will turn your teeth brown, so break out the whitening strips.

The tea does provide a nice little diversion from water now and again though. It seems to help with digestion, and in settling the stomach if you're feeling a little nauseous. If you like your tea sweet (for our friends in the South and from the British Isles), then may we humbly suggest that you *not* use regular sugar or artificial sweeteners. If it becomes a toss-up between artificial stuff or regular sugar, take the sugar every time.

Artificial sweeteners are incredibly bad for you. They actually break down in the body into formaldehyde (yes, the stuff that they embalm people with), and that formaldehyde does not break down further, but is actually stored in the brain. Many people suffer from terrible headaches and have found that when they stopped ingesting artificial sweeteners in any form (soda pop too) that their headaches virtually disappeared. My own sister and mother are two people for whom this has been true.

If you must sweeten things (and that's okay), we strongly suggest either brown sugar, honey, white sugar, or Splenda® which is made from sugar. Please remember that all of these contain extra calories, and sugar turns to glucose which when unused turns to stored fat in the body. You don't have to completely eliminate sugar, just be aware of how much and how often you ingest it.

Well, I guess that's about it for now. We really could have done a whole separate book on crazy little things like this, but we decided to let you find your own stuff to fill up your personal junk drawer. Along the way you'll discover your own unique oddities that work for you, and you'll be making notes for at least a year on these weird little experiences. As you do, just tuck them away in your mental junk drawer because just as in real life, no two junk drawers are the same, and they're each very specific to the home in which they reside.

So with that, this junk drawer is now full, and needs to be closed. The next time you need that odd but useful thing that doesn't seem to reside anywhere else, remember to check the junk drawer first.

SLAM!

Chapter Fourteen

SHRINK!

SHRANK!

SHRUNK!

Randal S. Baker M.D., F.A.C.S.
Julie M. Janeway
Karen J. Sparks

As the title states, you've had surgery to *shrink*, you *shrank* down to a more healthy weight, and now you've pretty much *shrunk* to the size you want to maintain. Can you conjugate the verb "to shrink? I bet you can if you try...." (Apologies to Mr. Rogers. He probably won't be my neighbor now that I've made fun of him.) So, now that you've been through this process, what's left is maintaining your new weight and healthy lifestyle, and dealing with a few other little issues and questions that might crop up.

One of the most commonly raised patient questions goes something like this: "What about all that extra, flabby, hangy-down skin after you lose the weight? Isn't that a big problem?" I usually respond, "If in one to two years you have extra, flabby-type skin hanging around, it is an excellent problem to have!" I say this not to be dismissive or insensitive, but to point out that the apparent cosmetic dislike of excessive skin pales in significance to the medical problems related to the morbid obesity you had in the first place.

In other words, by the time you have baggy skin (if you have it at all – a lot of patients do not have excess skin issues), many, if not most of your serious weight related medical problems will be significantly improved, and maybe even gone. Unlike obesity, baggy skin does not lead to diabetes, high blood pressure, heart disease, arthritis, sleep apnea, stroke, and an increased risk of some cancers. Many long for the day when the only problem they have to deal with is some "hangy-down" skin! Having plastic surgery to remove excess skin is not the automatic final step in the bariatric surgery process.

According to the American Society for Bariatric Surgery, in 2004 approximately 140,000 people had weight loss surgery in the United States alone, and the number is expected to more than double in 2005.[1] That was significantly more than had the surgery in 2003, and according to the American Society of Plastic Surgeons, more than 52,000 post-bariatric plastic surgery procedures were performed in 2003 (remembering that many patients had more than one plastic surgery procedure performed).[2]

The number of patients seeking plastic surgery for body contouring after dramatic weight loss is expected to increase by at least 20 percent in 2005 over the 2004 numbers, according to the American Society for Aesthetic Plastic Surgeons.[3]

Body contouring after bariatric surgery has become a field of special interest to many plastic surgeons, and they are beginning to realize that bariatric patients have different needs and issues than non-bariatric body contouring patients. Body contouring and shaping plastic surgery is more difficult for the post-bariatric surgery patient because the skin has generally been permanently damaged by being so extremely stretched. As a result of this stretching, patients' skin will generally loosen with age faster than patients who have not been obese, which may result in a degradation of the surgical results.[4]

Another issue for post-bariatric surgery patients having plastic surgery is controlling post-operative nausea and vomiting resulting from anesthetic and other medications. Excessive vomiting may cause ulceration of the pouch or esophagus, and may damage the connections in the new gastric anatomy. This can be controlled well for all patients, but especially for weight loss surgery patients, by administering an intravenous dose of anti-nausea medications before or during surgery. Bariatric patients seeking plastic surgery after full weight loss should locate a plastic surgeon who is familiar with the special needs of weight loss surgery patients.

All this being said, there is a legitimate role for plastic surgery after significant weight loss. Major weight gain puts tremendous strain on the entire body, including the skin and fascia. The skin becomes stretched and usually shows strain patterns (translation: stretch marks) similar to those seen on the abdomens of women after pregnancy. For persons who lose large amounts of weight, the skin often does not regain its original shape. For these people, plastic surgery becomes an option.

In addition, the older you are, the less resiliency in your skin. Many people who lose weight in their 20s and 30s do not have nearly as much wrinkled and excess skin. Often when they lose all of their excess weight it becomes difficult to know that they were ever obese. As a general rule: the older you are, the greater the likelihood of more excessive skin after weight loss. But remember, excessive skin is not solely the domain of the "mature." It can affect people who are not yet even in their twenties depending on how stretched the skin became during the term of obesity.

The most common excess skin issue deals with the fat and skin on the lower abdomen. Significant weight loss can leave a large hanging "apron" of excess skin and fat below the stomach area which is called a *panniculus*. In some patients this can be what many women call a little "poochy tummy," and can look relatively normal. In other patients, however, it can hang down to the thigh and knee area obstructing walking, can pull or inordinately strain lower back and abdominal muscles, can cause yeast infections or become infected, causes hygiene issues, and can create terrible difficulties with proper clothing fit.

Probably the second biggest complaint is flabby skin that may appear in the upper arms and thighs. Again, not all patients encounter this problem. Men in particular, tend not to have issues with their arms or thighs. The reality is, however, that if you are going to have excess skin in these areas, no amount of toning or weight lifting is going to completely eliminate it.

Whether it's the arms, the thighs, or the abdomen, the fascia (connective tissue) region of the muscles also becomes stretched with weight gain. Unfortunately, fascia does not shrink significantly after weight loss surgery, or after having a baby either for that matter. Just like arms and thighs, it's a mistake to think that "toning" or exercise will help shrink the fascia on the belly. If you have loose skin anywhere, you have only two choices: deal with it and be grateful you're no longer obese and unhealthy, or have it removed.

So, what's involved in having it removed? Well, surgery is sometimes medically recommended if the large "fatty apron" has infections and open sores, or interferes with daily activities such as walking. Usually though, surgery for excess skin is entirely cosmetic. As such, most insurance companies only cover surgery if it is deemed "medically necessary." Patients who desire plastic surgery often have to pay out of pocket, and plastic surgery is not cheap.

It is also important to note that plastic surgery involves the exchange of one cosmetic problem (loose skin) for another (scars). Most plastic surgeons will tell you that if you are unwilling to accept scars, you should not have plastic surgery as no surgeon can predict how the scars will heal on your body. Julie has told me many times that she would love to have some of the skin removed from her upper arms, but she is not willing to have to live with two more scars.

From past experience, Julie already knows that she scars badly, and to her, the excess skin is a small price to pay for the weight loss. Her arms are much smaller, she has no problem with clothing fit, and the skin is sound and causing no problems. Both she and I see no real need for plastic surgery on her arms. Does she have arms like Madonna? No. Does she need arms like Madonna? No. Is she healthy? YES.

For those determined to follow the plastic surgery path, however, there are a variety of surgeries available for the removal of excess skin and fat. The surgery that removes the excess panniculus, or skin and fat of the apron on the lower belly is called a *panniculectomy*. This surgery usually involves a large incision low on the abdomen where the excessive skin and fat are removed but the fascia is not touched. This is the type of surgery most likely to be covered, if at all, by your insurance company.

In contrast, an *abdominoplasty* includes removal of the excess skin and fat from the upper abdomen, along with tightening the fascia over the main muscle of the belly wall. Often times *liposuction* (suctioning of fat) is also done to contour the abdomen and waist line. This surgery gives a flatter appearance to the abdominal area and is often performed in conjunction with a panniculectomy (lower abdomen) in order to remove all the excess skin from the mid region of the torso.

These three surgeries together are sometimes referred to as a *mid-body lift*. Unfortunately, quite often this surgery is not covered by insurance, and patients are left to pay on their own. *Thigh lifts, arm lifts, facelifts,* and *total body lifts* can also be considered if necessary, but are almost always totally cosmetic and not covered by insurance.

A *medial thigh lift* is performed by making an incision along the inner thigh, and the location and length of the scar is based on the amount of skin that needs to be removed. Incisions can range from four inches, to the entire length of the thigh from the groin to just above the knee. Once the incision is made, the excess skin is removed, and the remaining skin is redraped over the muscles.

If a thigh or leg lift is performed in conjunction with an abdominoplasty, and a *butt lift*, it is referred to as a *lower body lift*. A lower body lift may or may not include liposuction as well. A medial thigh lift addresses the excess skin on the inside of the thighs, while a lower body lift addresses the excess skin on the front, back, and outer thighs.

A *butt lift*, sometimes referred to as a *gluteplasty* or *glutepexy* (top of the buttocks), or *excisional back lipidectomy* (bottom of the lower back), is exactly what you would imagine it to be. It is the procedure that removes skin from the upper gluteal (buttock) and/or lower back region in order to lift and tighten all the skin below it. This procedure has an added benefit in that it tends to raise the skin on the back of the thighs a bit as well. The scar for a butt lift generally extends across the entire backside from hip to hip.

Moving up the body from hip to breast, another problem many women encounter is *masto ptosis*, or *breast droop* following significant weight loss. Breast droop is defined as the situation in which the nipple has actually drooped below the crease beneath the breast. In situations where the nipple remains above the crest, and only breast tissue sags below the crest, it is referred to as a pseudo-droop.

Breast augmentation surgery, or *breast implants* will improve pseudo-droop, but will not usually do anything for women who have drooping breasts. For this problem, a *breast lift* or *mastopexy* is the procedure that may be needed. In a breast lift a key hole incision is made from the crest of the breast up and around the nipple. The nipple is moved up, and excess skin (and possibly fat) is removed. The breast incision is then closed, leaving an incision scar from the site of the new nipple placement down to the crest of the breast. An additional scar may appear across the crest of the breast depending on the size of the reduction that was performed, or if implants were placed. As a general rule, the more extensive the droop, the more extensive the scars.

If a patient develops excess skin in the upper arms, the only way to improve this problem is through an *arm lift*, or *brachioplasty*. The brachioplasty is done in a very similar fashion to the medial thigh lift. The major disadvantage of an arm lift is that the scars will extend down the length of the inside of the upper arm, from armpit to elbow. If you wear long sleeves to cover the excess skin on your arms, will you be forced to wear long sleeves to cover the scars on your arms? If so, then why put yourself through a surgical procedure, as all surgeries have the potential for complications and other issues? The advantages and disadvantages must always be weighed in determining whether or not to have plastic surgery. It can be very beneficial and affirming, but can also lead to the creation of other problems you could just as well do without.

Another issue many weight loss patients would rather do without is the problem of sagging skin on their faces or neck. Other excess skin issues can be covered by clothing, but sagging facial or neck skin is a real problem in that it can't really be covered, and it makes patients feel older and less attractive. Feeling better about yourself, your health, and your appearance are basic reasons for losing weight to begin with, so results that contradict that are often unacceptable to patients who have worked so hard to change their bodies.

A *face lift* or *rhytidectomy* will lift sagging cheeks, eliminate those pesky jowls, and contour the jawline. It can also remove excess fat under the chin or lift sagging skin on the neck. What it will not do, is eliminate wrinkles, sun damage, acne scars, and other skin issues. For those types of skin problems other procedures such as *dermabrasion, chemical peels,* and *laser resurfacing* may be available, and you should consult with a dermatologist or plastic surgeon. Sagging eyelids or foreheads can require different surgeries as well.

Face lift scars generally start above your ear, move down in front of your ear, and go behind the earlobe into the hairline. Another incision is made under the chin. Most scars fade quite well, and can be hidden with makeup. After three months or so, the scars are usually undetectable, although no surgeon can make that guarantee. Face lifts are one of the less invasive reconstructive procedures for bariatric patients, compared to procedures such as lower body lifts, and total body lifts that can place in the body 600 or more incision stitches during one operation.

Many of the plastic surgeries that are done on patients after weight loss surgery also involve *liposuction*. Liposuction is done two ways: *tumescent* and *ultrasonic*. Tumescent, or *true tumescent* liposuction is the type of fat suctioning surgery that has been performed in the United States since the 1970s. This form of liposuction involves filling the fat with tumescent fluid (saline with adrenaline and lidocaine) to make the fat stiffer, and reduce bleeding and discomfort.

Once the fat has been stiffened by the tumescent liquid, it is then suctioned out by the insertion of long thin rods called cannulas. The tiny incisions involved are often hidden in skin creases, and are generally no bigger than the incisions made for laparoscopic bariatric surgery.

Ultrasonic liposuction on the other hand, involves the infusion of tumescent fluid to stiffen the fat, but rather than suctioning the stiffened fat out in its globular form, the surgeon uses an ultrasonic rod (energy waves similar to sound, but higher frequencies) to liquify the fat before it is removed. The rod is inserted through tiny incisions as well. As it passes by the fat it liquefies it, and it is then suctioned out in a fluid form.

Plastic surgery professionals are split over the issue of which technique is better. Although both techniques have a very low incidence of blood loss to begin with, there is slightly less blood loss with ultrasonic. Discomfort seems to be about equal for both. The best advice we can give you is to consult with your plastic surgeon on which technique is right for you. Plastic surgeons will usually recommend the technique with which they are most familiar and that is always a plus for the patient, unless you are willing to volunteer to be the patient on which they learn a new technique.

For weight loss surgery patients in general, it is best to wait at least one, to one and a half years post-bariatric procedure before considering any type of plastic surgery. Patients fare far better when they wait for their weight to stabilize, because their bodies are healthier going into surgery. Patients who wait for plastic surgery experience fewer infections, respiratory complications, and wound reopenings. Those who forge ahead with premature surgery will often desire to have the surgery repeated because of further laxity of the skin as a result of further weight loss.

Generally plastic surgery is not medically necessary, and there is no real rush to get into it. Many patients do not choose to pursue this type of surgery, and that option is fine as well. The goal is to learn to live as realistic and normal a life as possible, with as few surgical interventions as possible.

With that said, I believe a word about realistic expectations is needed at this juncture. Plastic surgery will help some with overall appearance and self-acceptance but don't expect the "extreme makeover" hype as seen in many television shows. You are not likely going to look like Barbie Beauty after surgery if you didn't resemble her before. And guess what? You don't need to! You are fine being you.

The most important thing is that you are no longer suffering from obesity, have improved or resolved its serious related medical conditions, and you are now much more healthy and vital than you were before. It has been my experience that some patients are just not happy with themselves in general, and keep looking toward plastic surgery (and even bariatric surgery) to make a fairy tale ending to a not-so fairy tale life. These expectations are often hollow and lead to disappointment.

Like any other surgery, plastic surgery has risks: some significant, and some not so significant. These must be realistically discussed with your surgeon prior to any attempt at "reconstruction" or "body contouring." Just keep in mind that the excess skin dilemma is a not-so-bad circumstance to find oneself in after claiming a total success and victory over morbid obesity.

Additionally, maintenance is key to long-term success with plastic surgery as well as bariatric surgery. Unhealthy eating and little exercise will challenge and reverse some of the best plastic surgery results. As noted repeatedly in this book, a total lifestyle change will be necessary to achieve the best result possible.

Keeping up the habits you developed to get the weight off, and continually developing new and better ones is what the maintenance portion is all about. If you think it's just going to stay off, you're wrong. You'll have to work at it like everybody else, for the rest of your life.

Keep your life in perspective and appreciate it every day, even when the days are tough for whatever reason. Remind yourself that balance is a new life credo. Balance all things: food, exercise, self-concept, work, attitude, ego, etc. Don't go overboard on any one thing. This metamorphosis was designed to give you a good start on a good life, now it's up to you to maintain it. It was not designed to move you off in any one direction so far as to become completely unrecognizable in any aspect from the person who started the journey.

Periodically take photographs of yourself, and really look at them. Make sure that you're not just seeing what you want to see in the mirror, or what your mind wants to see as being you. Make sure you aren't putting the weight back on. Make sure that you aren't turning yourself into someone you're not, like trying to reclaim lost youth by sporting clothing your thirteen year old daughter wears!

Being your age, whatever it is, is okay. Celebrate the fact that you have lived, and given your previous weight circumstances, that you have survived those years. Be glad for the knowledge, wisdom, insight, experiences, and love you have felt through those years. Be happy with what you have accomplished, and don't fixate on what you have missed. There's nothing more pathetic than someone in their thirties (or later), male or female, trying to act and dress like they are still in their early twenties (or worse yet, teens!).

It's okay to feel young. It's okay to act as a vital, alive person. But remember to be who you are and make the most out of what is happening now, not waste it trying to relive lost years or opportunities. Put the past in the past. Embrace the here-and-now, and look excitedly toward the future. You deserve it!

Make it a rule of life never to regret

and never to look back.

Regret is an appalling waste of energy;

you can't build on it;

it is only good for wallowing in.

KATHERINE MANSFIELD

Chapter Fifteen

THE FINAL BATTLE:
⤙ DEFEAT ⤚
OF THE CLONES

Randal S. Baker M.D., F.A.C.S.

You've made it to the end of this book, and that means we've pretty thoroughly explored weight loss surgery, one particular method of dealing with obesity. Surgery is the most effective means available today for dealing with the disease and its related maladies. But what about in the future? How will obesity be treated, or possibly eliminated in the future? Will we really have to live for another fifty or one hundred years putting up with all those obnoxious miracle-diet commercials that are simply clones of each other? Will the miracle-diet clones take over the airwaves of the future? Good Heavens, we hope not!

More than likely the future will *not* be populated with a growing profusion of miracle-diet clones claiming to cure obesity and "whatever else ails ya!" I have no doubt, however, that these clones will continue to exist in some form or another as the age old tradition of "snake oil" sales seems to defy time, space, and social progress. Sadly, the clones will co-exist for a little while at least, while advances in varying technologies aimed at defeating obesity (and hopefully defeating the miracle-diet clones as well!) continue to evolve.

The future will likely see several diverse approaches to treating and/or eliminating the obesity epidemic. As the cause is essentially a combination of genetic predispositions and environment, scientists will have to combat the issue on both fronts. At present the surgical battle-plan offers a way to "fool" the genetic predispositions, and force some environmental changes. Less food makes one feel full, overeating leads to nausea and vomiting, and eating the wrong foods can lead to dumping (auto eject). The weapon is an effective one, but isn't available to all combatants in the battle.

Currently, surgery is only recommended for patients in the *morbidly obese* camp (BMI greater than 40), because the risk/benefit ratio is not as medically justifiable for people in the *overweight* and *obese* categories (BMI between 25 and 39). Remember that approximately 65% of the U.S. population is *overweight* and *obese*, and that number is increasing dramatically, but the surgical option is not generally available to them in their battle with the bulge.

I believe that improvements will continue to make surgery safer, as well as to possibly open up the field for the use of less-invasive surgical techniques (laparoscopic RYGB or Lap-Band®) for patients even in the *obese* category. The use of less invasive "micro-surgical" techniques on patients in all obesity related categories may even become commonplace in the future battle to win the war on weight.

We may also see the development of surgical and non-surgical products designed to provide fullness and encourage weight loss. Currently, a device called an *implantable gastric stimulator* is being tested in the United States. This device, more commonly referred to by researchers as a *gastric pacemaker*, is about the size of a matchbox. It is surgically implanted under the skin of the abdomen, and a connecting wire is implanted in the wall of the stomach. The device aims at emitting electrical pulses to the stomach muscles to create a feeling of fullness. It is hoped that this feeling of fullness will then cause the patient to eat less.

The pacemaker's electrical emissions create a feeling of fullness by slowing down the process of peristalsis, and making the patient feel full with less in the stomach. The mechanism is not unlike the decreased empting of the stomach that occurs with the stomach flu. Signing up for permanent "stomach flu" may not be most people's idea of a good way to lose weight. In addition, results have been sporadic, and complications like gastric perforation, lead dislodgement, pain, nausea, and vomiting are not infrequent. The amount of weight lost with pacing is significantly less than with present bariatric surgeries. Ultimately, the question remains whether the technology will be helpful for those in the obese category, for whom surgery is presently not an option.

The gastric pacemaker has received approvals in several European countries and Canada, and is currently in clinical trials in the United States. Studies in other countries have shown that patients typically lose only around 25 percent of their excess weight, but such a loss will still have a positive effect on their health. Preliminary results of a multicenter, randomized, controlled, double-blind study in the U.S. showed in its preliminary results no significant difference in weight loss with the pacing stimulated vs. nonstimulated patient participants.

No data presently exists on the long-term efficacy or safety of this device. Our suspicions are that absent multidisciplinary measures to address all causative factors of obesity, the device will not show significant permanent weight reductions for patients employing it. Also, more time and study will also be needed to assess any possible untoward effects of the electrical stimulation on other parts of the body. As it requires surgery, (not unlike RYGB or Lap-Band® procedures), and all surgeries carry risks, the risk to benefit ratio for the morbidly obese still seems to favor the current weight loss surgeries over the gastric pacemaker device.

All of these potential devices, applications, and procedures should be offered through comprehensive, multidisciplinary centers that can care for all of the weight related changes (medication, dietary, behavioral, and exercise related), which ensue with obesity and weight loss. None of the surgical or non-surgical options will work in isolation, so the nutrition, behavioral, and exercise issues must be addressed as well.

As the invasive nature of the procedures and the attendant potential complications decrease, we may see more surgical application not only for people who are significantly less than *morbidly obese*, but also for children and adolescents as well. The obesity epidemic in children and adolescents is already at an all-time high. This demographic is where we really need to aim our efforts in order to halt the overwhelming advance toward obesity, and cut it off at its root source.

With regard to the awareness of childhood obesity, the future is beginning now. Various countries around the world have begun to look seriously at the weight and health of their nations' children, and to assess the potential long-range ramifications on the economy and social structure of their nations as a result of the epidemic.

Indeed, many U.S. states have Bills that are pending, or been recently passed that are aimed at addressing the childhood obesity problem. From cracking down on the poor nutritional content of school lunch programs, to increased, mandatory daily physical education requirements, states are looking long and hard at the weighty matter of heavy kids.

The other main way to affect this epidemic is by a major change on the environmental side of the equation. Television, computers, and video games have resulted in less physical activity in children, fewer calories burned, and more pounds being carried. A new generation of games and toys, however, could possibly begin to reverse this trend.

In fact, Julie was telling me just the other day about another physician friend of hers, Dr. Edmond Ducommun, who has been working with a neuropsychologist colleague on a device that would be implanted in children's shoes, much like the device that makes the little light in their athletic shoes light up when they walk. The device won't make their shoes glow, but it will keep track of how many steps they take.

The device then relays the message to a storage unit that is worn on the wrist and doubles as a watch. The "watch" tallies the steps and converts the total number of steps involved into credits that are used for time spent on the computer, television, gaming station, or DVD/VCR player. The watch transmits the accumulated credits to receivers attached to these components, thereby limiting little Johnny's use of them, and encouraging him to run around and play more so he can play his video game again later.

Now, I know what you're thinking, and I thought it too: "How are you going to keep the kid from just sitting there banging the shoe repeatedly while he's watching the television in order to rack up more credits?" Well, apparently they've thought of that, and have built in some safeguard that involves some major formula referencing weight, pressure, impact, torque, velocity, mass, and a bunch of other physics-type things that involve way too much math.

I also asked what would happen if Johnny didn't have enough credits to watch T.V., and came into the room while Susie was watching it on her credits. Would the T.V. turn off to prevent Johnny from getting a free ride? They claim to have thought of that as well and have some system in place that will prevent one device from canceling out another. It will purportedly work on the same system used to prevent one keyless entry remote from opening all cars of a similar make parked in the area, or preventing all the garage doors in the subdivision from going up or down at the same time when you press your door opener remote. I guess if Susie is watching and Johnny sits down to watch too, the safeguard for that is still parental supervision.

This product has already been proto-typed, is patent-pending, and is now in the design enhancement process. It's just one of many new products being created to get kids back outside and moving like they should be. It can be put into almost anything: a basketball, on a bike, on a free weight, on a tennis racquet, or on a baseball bat. If you want to measure the movement force of something, it can be incorporated. The possibilities are almost endless. Maybe it will be the big "must-have" item for parents for the 2008 Holiday season.

For now, we just need to encourage kids to be active and play outside more often (weather and other conditions permitting). My kids recently received a laser tag game with which they stampede throughout the house (more than usual), chasing each other with laser guns and helmets. The house and furniture have taken a beating, but the kids are getting good exercise and having fun in the process.

For those of you in Florida or Arizona wondering why my kids are cavorting inside the house, just remember we have two basic seasons in Michigan: Winter (the longest), and road construction (the harshest). At present, it's Winter, but we've seen orange barrels beginning to sprout, so construction must be just around the corner!

If we are to properly treat the obesity epidemic in the future, an overall emphasis on more activity will be essential to help restructure the present obesity encouraging environmental conditions. In fact, by the year 2030, daily life might just sound a little like this:

> "Where's Jason?" Devin asked. "He's playing his 'Exploring Mars' game in the virtual reality room," Rebecca replied. "He's been at it since he came home from school. He has about 15 more minutes until he reaches his exercise requirement credits for today, but I suspect that he'll be in there until we call him for dinner. He loves that new game, but he keeps whining that the Martian landscape is too steep, and he gets tired of climbing before he can close in on the lost treasure."
>
> Devin thought a minute and said, "I don't know what he's whining about, when we were kids we had to drive ten miles, up hill, both ways, in the blinding snow, and biting cold, with no heated seats, just to get to a friend's house so we could sit in the basement, eat cheese puffs, and play video games! These kids just don't know how easy they have it with balanced meals and snacks, interactive 3-D games, and climate controlled environments. We were forced to sit on the basement floor for a million hours a year playing stupid, unrealistic games. They can play games in whatever climate and conditions they want, they aren't forced to ruin their backs and posture like we were, and their snacks not only taste good, but are good for them too! Kids today take everything for granted!"

If this is the future, then some things will never change! In addition to emphasis on increased exercise, better nutrition, and surgical interventions, pharmaceutical breakthroughs may also be seen, but these will likely be expensive and plagued with side effects. Recently, I heard a report about the newly discovered hormone, *ghrelin*. It has been found that ghrelin is higher in thin people and lower in obese people.[1] In fact, researchers have discovered that after gastric bypass ghrelin levels drop, so now the race is on to find a drug to block this hormone.[2] During one of the studies of a potential drug to inhibit ghrelin production, they discovered that ghrelin is actually also involved in memory.[3] The rats did lose weight but they didn't know it, and they couldn't remember where they lived, who each other were, or how to get back to the cage! So there you go.

All medications have side effects and/or adverse effects. Many of these side effects do not become apparent until wide spread usage is engaged. (Take Celebrex® and Phen-fen® as examples.) Although the pharmaceutical industry will probably want to assail me with literature to the contrary, I think the major effective obesity break-throughs will not be in this area. The "in your face" quick fix miracle-diet clones will not likely be significantly thwarted by any pharmaceutical advances either. They'll simply pick up on some of the "junk science" and spin it into another clone offering a miracle cure for your weight problems.

Another area of potential, if not eventual success, is related to gene therapy. According to geneticists, more than one gene is responsible for obesity. It is thought that there are many gene sequences that predispose humans toward obesity.[4] To be able to "fix" these genetic sequences would be a huge breakthrough, but we're prob-ably not going to see that for some time. A lot of miracle-diet clones will prevail before this research area comes through with a decent arsenal of weapons ready to do battle in the weight wars, and defeat the miracle-diet clones.

Gene therapy will represent a breakthrough for multiple medical maladies not just obesity, but unfortunately it is a long way off. Perhaps, gene therapy might affect the future somewhat like this:

> *Lucas passed through the antiviral decontaminator and paused briefly as the detection unit identified another mutated avian virus that somehow got on his clothes. After decontamination he entered the kitchen and called out "Laura, I'm home. How did the doctor's visit go?" Laura came into the kitchen and said, "It went great. The baby is doing well, but the genetic sequence screen identified dysfunc-tional leptin and alpha-ghrelin related genes, which will predispose little Mary Beth or Noah for obesity. It also found some other pro-pancreatic cancer sequence thingy, and the genetic sequence for heart disease. On the walk home I stopped and set up an appointment for a G.O.N.E procedure (genetic outpatient neomalgene eradicator) to correct the problems." "That's good. At least they didn't find anything significant," Lucas replied.*

The year 2030 may not even be far enough in the future for us to see the use of genetic correction therapy, so until then the current methods of preventing obesity through good nutrition and exercise will have to suffice.

Speaking of nutrition, however, I expect that the future will see an increased emphasis being placed on eating a more balanced diet, and reducing the amount of saturated fat, trans fat, sugar, and grease we consume. We're already seeing a trend toward better nutrition, even in the fast food industry. We're seeing wrap sandwiches that eliminate much of the breads used in regular sandwiches, more salads are being offered with dressings that have lower fat content, and fruit is even appearing in many fast food restaurants for both children and adults to help balance our diets.

Ensuring a good balanced diet requires work, and the work is made more complex by the fast paced lives we live. We rarely have our meals together as families anymore, and trying to control all nutrition sources, especially in our children's lives is difficult. Until we develop a program for the computers in our "smart homes" to keep track of our caloric intake and exercise, we need to have some significant "work arounds" to help us stay fit and healthy.

We and our children need to learn how to go into a restaurant and not come out having been "bigger sized." Draconian "diets" do not work as no one can stand the monotony of the featured foods, or the deprivation of foods that taste good for long periods of time. And, as we've concluded, miracle-diet clones are nothing but "snake oil" in a new package.

A basic balanced approach with an emphasis on proper types of food and overall calories ingested will be necessary for long-term success. We need to learn and apply that knowledge now, and teach it consistently and regularly to our children so we can keep them from having to worry about dealing with weight problems. For our children, going to school and memorizing the food pyramid while eating snack cakes and chips at lunch and not having the most important food groups from the pyramid in the school and home is a recipe for defeat. Defeat in this instance, is equivalent to fat and weight gain.

Emphasis on creating good tasting food choices from the base of the food pyramid should be stressed. Today many of the important food groups are mostly available as tasteless cardboard consistency gruel. Most healthy whole grain cereals taste like gravel with sand thrown in. And most of these "healthy" cereals have boxes with boring nutrition facts and insipid graphics that probably taste better than the contents. If I have to eat gravel, at least let me look at exciting puzzles and cartoons to keep my mind off the taste and texture! Grape Nuts® could learn a thing or two from Fruit Loops®, and vice versa.

In addition to good tasting healthy foods, and amusing packaging to help us eat better, perhaps the future will bring us technologies to track our nutritional consumption as well. It may be a unit linked to the computers that will automate our homes, or maybe it will be hand-held like a PDA, I don't know. Maybe the future will be a little like this:

Haleigh yelled, "Honey, I'm home! What's for dinner? I'm starving!" Jordan laughed as he took Courtney's school bag off the couch and put it at the bottom of the stairs, "When aren't you starving? I've been busy all day with a conference call to Tokyo, so I set the Cookmaster to 'auto chef'" said Jordan. "It says it planned a special tuna and rice dish to completely balance this week's food pyramid program. Courtney and I even get some dessert tonight because we haven't used all our simple carbohydrate quotas for the week. Courtney can actually have seconds on dessert because the school lunch program has an even more restrictive carb quota than we do, but I'm not telling her that!" Haleigh groaned; tuna casserole again.

"Do I get dessert?" she asked. "No, because you keep eating fast food for lunch, and you're way over your carb quota for the week. If you'd let the Cookmaster prepare your lunch and take it with you to work, maybe you could eat dessert when you got home," said Jordan. "The next time you're at the drive thru maybe you should 'small size' your order from the healthwise menu, and eat less junk food on your breaks," Jordan added. Haleigh, nodded her head in agreement, and said, "I'll start on that tomorrow, but for tonight I'm eating Courtney's extra dessert. What she doesn't know won't hurt her!"

Not only is personal responsibility for proper nutrition and exercise essential, but an overall emphasis by entire communities is necessary as well. Effective education and real programs with results are needed, not just symbolic "feel good" seminars. Recently, I attended such a meeting where a well-meaning and well-intentioned group presented its "child first" weight control program.

The program focused mainly on the emotional side of the issue. I support treating this part of the problem entirely, as self-loathing is a defeatist behavior, and poor self-esteem feeds the cycle of eating and self-loathing. But, it's only one component of the entire issue, and a comprehensive multi-disciplinary approach is essential to long-term success.

A peronalized action plan for weight management, modification of inappropriate eating behaviors, and monitored compliance with nutrition and exercise components were not being addressed at all. As a result of this approach, the kids were, unfortunately, still gaining unhealthy weight, but at least they felt better about themselves while doing so. I know it sounds like I am skewering some sacred cows or being anti-politically correct, but these feel good symbolic gestures are NOT working!

We need substance over symbolism to repulse obesity and those obnoxious miracle-diet clones. We need real action and real treatment, not just some well-intentioned band-aid being placed over a gaping chest wound! Obesity is a disease, and is best treated through prevention before symptoms occur. In this case, prevention isn't worth a pound of cure, it's worth a mountain range of cure!

In the mean time, as society's weight problems continue to increase, we really need to focus our collective attention on both obesity cure and prevention. We need a laser-fine focus that will begin to dramatically change the future of obesity as a disease and epidemic, and finally win the war on weight. Only then will all the quick fix miracle-diet clones really be vanquished, as true and lasting healthy lifestyles emerge. Alas, I fear it won't come soon enough. Until then... I still have some of my famous lemon extract for sale.

Chapter Sixteen

━ ADDITIONAL RESOURCES ━

Julie M. Janeway
Karen J. Sparks

The organizations, agencies, and web sites presented here were selected based on the value of the information presented on obesity, being overweight, weight loss treatments, and related conditions. The appearance in this chapter of any organization, agency, or web site, (or any products, programs, or services they may advertise or offer), does not constitute an endorsement by the publisher, MMPC®, MMPC® Center for Health Excellence, or any of the main or contributing authors of this book. While the information in these resources and web sites may be useful to those contemplating a weight loss program, anyone wishing to do so should consult a skilled bariatric physician or surgeon.

• Indicates site has a physician locator service

Michigan Medical PC® — Center for Health Excellence
4100 Lake Drive, SE, Suite B01
Grand Rapids, MI 49546
(616) 974-4400
1-877-877-MMPC Toll Free
www.mmpc.com (click on Center for Health Excellence)

American Diabetes Association
1701 North Beauregard Street
Alexandria, VA 22311
(800) DIABETES (800-342-2383)
www.diabetes.org

The American Diabetes Association is the nation's leading nonprofit health organization providing diabetes research, information, and advocacy. The mission of the organization is to prevent and cure diabetes, and to improve the lives of all people affected by diabetes.

American Dietetic Association
120 S. Riverside Plaza, Suite 2000
Chicago, IL 60606-6995
(312) 877-1600
www.eatright.com

The American Dietetic Association promotes optimal nutrition, health, and well-being for all persons, as well as advocating for its membership comprised mainly of registered dietitians and nutritionists.

American Heart Association
7272 Greenville Avenue
Dallas, TX 75231
(800) AHA-USA1 (800-242-8721)
www.americanheart.org

The American Heart Association is a national voluntary health agency whose mission is to reduce disability and death from cardiovascular diseases and stroke.

American Medical Association (AMA)
515 North State Street
Chicago, IL 60610
(800) 621-8335
www.ama-assn.org

Founded more than 150 years ago, AMA's strategic agenda remains rooted in its historic commitment to standards, ethics, excellence in medical education and practice, and advocacy on behalf of the medical profession and the patients it serves.

American Obesity Association
1250 24th Street, NW, Suite 300
Washington, DC 20037
(800) 98-OBESE (800-986-2372)
www.obestiy.org

This association champions the cause of eliminating obesity by promoting education, research, and community action that can improve the quality of life and self-image of sufferers.

American Society for Aesthetic Plastic Surgery (ASAPS) *
36 W 44th Street, Suite 630
New York, NY 10036
(212) 921-0500
www.surgery.org

Founded in 1967, ASAPS is the leading professional organization of plastic surgeons certified by the American Board of Plastic Surgery who specialize in cosmetic plastic surgery.

American Society for Bariatric Physicians *
2821 S. Parker Road, Suite 625
Aurora, CO 80014
(303) 770-2526
www.asbp.org

The American Society of Bariatric Physicians is an international association of allied health care professionals with special interest and experience in the comprehensive treatment of overweight, obesity, and related disorders. Their purpose is to establish and maintain practice guidelines, and provide education to their members, the health care industry, and the public.

American Society for Bariatric Surgery (ASBS) *
1100 S.W. 75th Drive, Suite 201
Gainesville, FL 32607
(352) 331-4900
www.asbs.org

Founded in 1983, ASBS is the largest society in the world for this medical specialty. Many of the specialty's foremost American surgeons comprise this society's leadership, and have established an excellent organization with educational and support programs for surgeons and allied health professionals.

Association of Morbid Obesity Support *
P.O. Box 1504
Oakley, CA 94561-1504
(800) WLS-INFO (800-957-4636)
www.obestiyhelp.com

Founded in 1998, obesityhelp.com is dedicated to the education, empowerment, and support of all individuals affected by obesity, along with all others (friends, employers, physicians, etc.) concerned. It focuses on common people afflicted with this common problem. Though technically a corporation, their focus is explicitly peer-to-peer oriented, and non-commercial in nature. They aspire to defeat ignorance, isolation, and discrimination against the clinical disease of obesity.

Centers for Disease Control and Prevention (CDC)
1600 Clifton Road
Atlanta, GA 30333
(404) 639-3534 (800) 311-3435
www.cdc.gov

The Centers for Disease Control and Prevention (CDC) is recognized as the leading federal agency for protecting the health and safety of people – at home and abroad – by providing credible information to enhance health decisions, and promoting health through strong partnerships. The CDC serves as the national focus for developing and applying disease prevention and control, environmental health, and health promotion and education activities designed to improve the health of the people of the United States.

CBS Health Watch
www.cbsnews.com/sections/health/main204.shtml

Medscape takes consumer health information to a new level with CBS Health Watch, which offers an array of high-quality information and interactive tools to help consumers and their families manage their daily personal health.

Ethicon Endo-Surgery, Inc.
4545 Creek Road
Cincinnati, OH 45242
1-800-USE-ENDO
www.weightlosssurgeryinfo.com

Ethicon Endo-Surgery is a Johnson & Johnson company dedicated to helping patients find and understand credible information about weight loss surgery options and procedures.

International Bariatric Surgery Registry
Dept. of Surgery, University of Iowa Hospitals & Clinics
200 Hawkins Drive, 1504 JCP
Iowa City, IA 52242-1086
(800) 777-8442
halsted.surgery.uiowa.edu/ibsr

The purpose of the IBSR is to promote optimum care of patients undergoing surgical treatments for severe obesity, and to give medical providers standardized clinical data collection and analysis.

National Eating Disorders Association
Eating Disorders Awareness and Prevention, Inc.
603 Stewart Street, Suite 803
Seattle, WA 98101
(206) 382-3587
www.edap.org

EDAP is the nation's largest nonprofit organization devoted to the awareness and treatment of eating disorders.

National Heart, Lung, and Blood Institute (National Institutes of Health)
NHLBI Information Center
P.O. Box 30105
Bethesda, MD 20824-0105
(301) 592-8573
www.nhlbi.nih.gov

The National Heart, Lung, and Blood Institute (NHLBI) provides leadership for a national program in diseases of the heart, blood vessels, lung, blood, blood resources, and sleep disorders. The Institute plans, conducts, fosters, and supports an integrated and coordinated program of basic research, clinical investigations and trials, observational studies, demonstrations, and educational projects.

The National Institutes of Health (NIH)
9000 Rockville Pike
Bethesda, MD 20892
(301) 496-4000
www.nih.gov

Founded in 1887, the National Institutes of Health is one of the world's foremost medical research centers. It is comprised of 25 separate institutes and centers, all part of the U.S. Department of Health and Human Services.

North American Association for the Study of Obesity *
8630 Fenton Street, Suite 918
Silver Spring, MD 20910
(301) 563-6526
www.naaso.org

The North American Association for the Study of Obesity is an interdisciplinary scientific society dedicated to the study of obesity. They are committed to encouraging research on the causes and treatment of obesity, and to keeping the medical community and public informed of new advances.

Sleepnet.com *
www.sleepnet.com

This is an educational web site that provides visitors with information on sleep disorders, terms and definitions, tips for better sleep, as well as useful links to other well rated informational web sites.

The Surgeon General's Call to Action to Prevent and Decrease Overweight and Obesity 2001
www.surgeongeneral.gov/topics/obesity

The Skinny Daily Post
www.skinnydaily.blogspot.com

Short daily essays on weight loss and fitness from people who have been there, done that, and work hard every day to keep their weight off.

WebMD
my.webmd.com/health_and_wellness/food_nutrition/lose_weight/default.htm

WebMD provides connectivity and a full suite of services to the healthcare industry that improve administrative efficiencies and clinical effectiveness enabling high-quality patient care.

Weight-Control Information Network (National Institute of Diabetes and Digestive and Kidney Disorders at the National Institutes of Health)
1 WIN Way
Bethesda, MD 20892-3665
(202) 828-1025 1-877-946-4627
www.niddk.nih.gov

The Weight-Control Information Network (WIN) is a national information service of the National Institute of Diabetes and Digestive and Kidney Disease (NIDDK), National Institutes of Health (NIH). WIN was established in 2004 to provide health professionals and consumers with science-based information on obesity, weight control, and motivation.

Chapter Seventeen

➤ GLOSSARY OF TERMS ➤

Abdominal cavity – The abdomen or abdominal cavity contains all of the digestive organs.

Absorption – Process by which digested food is absorbed by the lower part of the small intestine into the bloodstream.

Adhesions – The process of adhering or uniting two surfaces or parts, especially the union of the opposing surfaces of a wound. Inflammatory bands that connect opposing serous surfaces.

Adipose – Fatty; pertaining to fat.

Anemia – A decrease in hemoglobin in the blood to levels below the normal range of 12-16 g/dL for women and 13.5-18 g/dL for men. Anemia may be caused by a decrease in red cell production, an increase in red cell destruction, or a loss of blood.

Anastomosis – Surgical connection between two structures.

Anesthesia – Loss of sensation resulting from pharmacologic depression of nerve function or from neurological dysfunction.

Antihistamine – Any substance capable of reducing the physiologic and pharmacologic effects of histamine release in the body in response to allergic inflammatory reactions.

Bariatric – Pertaining to weight or weight reduction.

BMI-Body Mass Index – Method of calculating degree of excess weight. Based on weight and body surface area.

Bowel obstruction – Blocking or clogging of any portion of the bowel.

Calcium – An alkaline earth metal element. The fifth most abundant element in the human body, mainly present in the bone.

Cardiac dysfunction – Pertains to a heart that is unable to function normally; may also pertain to abnormality in function of the esophageal opening of the cardiac portion of the stomach.

Cardiovascular – Pertaining to heart and blood vessels.

Clinically severe obesity – Body Mass Index of 40 or more, which is roughly equivalent to 100 pounds or more over ideal body weight. Also known as Morbid Obesity.

Cognitive dissonance – A state of tension resulting from a discrepancy in a person's emotional and intellectual frame of reference for interpreting and coping with his or her environment. It usually occurs when new information contradicts existing assumptions or knowledge.

Colon – Large intestine beginning at the end of the small intestine and ending at the rectum.

Co-Morbidity – Illness (i.e., arthritis, hypertension) or disabling conditions associated with clinically severe obesity or obesity-related health conditions.

Congestive heart failure (CHF) – Heart failure in which the heart is unable to maintain an adequate circulation of blood in the bodily tissues or to pump out the venous blood returned to it by the veins.

Contraindications – Any symptom or circumstance indicating the inappropriateness of an otherwise advisable treatment (i.e., alcoholism; drug dependency; severe depression; sociopathic (antisocial) personality disorder).

Contrast swallow study – An x-ray that is performed to pinpoint problems that exist in a patient who is unable to swallow using a contrast medium which is a substance injected into the body via a catheter, or swallowed to facilitate radiographic imaging of structures and tissues.

Coronary artery disease (CAD) – The abnormal condition that may affect the heart's arteries and produce various pathologic effects, especially the reduced flow of oxygen and nutrients to the myocardium.

Criteria – Defines potential candidate for surgery treatment.

CT – Abbreviation for computed tomography. A radiographic technique that produces an image of a detailed cross section of tissue. It is a painless, noninvasive, test that requires no preparation.

Deep vein thrombosis (DVT) – A disorder involving a blood clot in one of the deep veins of the body, most commonly the iliac or femoral vein.

Degenerative joint disease – Inflammation of the joint which causes degenerative changes.

Digestion – Process by which food is broken down by the stomach and upper small intestine into absorbable forms.

Dilation – Process of enlarging a passage or anastomosis.

Dilatation – See dilation.

Disease – A condition of abnormal vital function involving any structure, part, or system of an organism. A specific illness or disorder characterized by a recognizable set of signs and symptoms, attributable to heredity, infection, diet, or environment. A process injurious to health and/or longevity.

Distention – The state of being swollen or expanded.

Diuretic – A drug or other substance tending to promote the formation and excretion of urine.

Dumping syndrome – Uncomfortable feeling of nausea, lightheadedness, upset stomach, diarrhea, associated with ingestion of sweets, high-calorie liquids, high fat foods, or dairy products.

Duodenum – First twelve inches of small intestine immediately below stomach. Bile and pancreatic fluids flow into the duodenum through ducts from the liver and pancreas respectively. This is where much of the iron and calcium is absorbed.

EGD – Abbreviation for esophagogastroduodenoscopy. An endoscopic examination of the esophagus, stomach, and duodenum.

EKG – Abbreviaton for electrocardiograph; a device used for recording the electrical activity in the myocardium to detect transmission of the cardiac impulse through the conductive tissues of the muscle. EKG allows diagnosis of specific cardiac abnormalities.

Electrolytes – An element or compound that when melted or dissolved in water or another solvent, dissociates into ions and is able to carry an electrical current. Proper quantities of principal electrolytes and balance among them are critical to normal metabolism and function.

Endoscopy – The visualization of the interior of organs and cavities of the body with an endoscope.

Esophagus – The esophagus is a long muscular tube, which moves food from the mouth to the stomach.

Flatulence – The presence of an excessive amount of air or gas in the stomach and intestinal tract, causing distention of the organs, and in some cases mild to moderate pain before exiting through the rectum.

Foley catheter – A rubber catheter (tube) with a balloon tip to be filled with a sterile liquid after it has been placed in the bladder. This kind of catheter is used when continuous drainage of the bladder is desired such as in surgery.

Folic acid – A yellow crystalline water-soluble vitamin essential for cell growth and reproduction.

Gastric – Pertaining to the stomach.

Gastroesophageal reflux disease – A back flow of contents of the stomach into the esophagus that is often the result of incompetence of the lower esophageal muscle. Gastric juices are acid and therefore produce burning pain in the esophagus.

Gastrointestinal tract – Pertaining to the stomach or intestine.

Gastrojejunostomy anastomosis – Upper connection of the Gastric Bypass operation.

Genetic – Pertains to transmitted hereditary characteristics.

Gestalt – A single physical, psychological, or symbolic configuration, pattern, or experience that consists of a number of elements and has an effect as a whole different from that of the sum of its parts.

HDL cholesterol – Abbreviation for high-density lipoprotein. HDL is a plasma protein made mainly in the liver and is involved in transporting cholesterol to the liver to be disposed.

Hemoglobin – A complex protein-iron compound in the blood that carries oxygen to the cells from the lungs and carbon dioxide away from the cells to the lungs.

Heparin – A naturally occurring substance that acts in the body as an anticlotting factor to prevent intervascular clotting.

Hernia – A weakness in the abdominal wall resulting in a detectable bulge.

Herniation – Process in which a hernia is formed.

Hyperlipidemia – High cholesterol. An excessive level of blood fats.

Hyperosmolality – Presence of highly concentrated substances capable of producing dumping syndrome.

Hypertension – High blood pressure.

Hypotension – Low blood pressure.

Hypothyroidism – An underfunctioning thyroid gland.

Hypoventilation syndrome – An abnormal condition of the respiratory system in which the volume of air that enters the lungs and takes part in the gas exchange is not adequate for the body's needs.

IFSO – International Federation for the Surgery of Obesity

Ileum – The last ten feet of small intestine; responsible for the absorption of fat-soluble vitamins A, D, E and K and other nutrients.

Ileus – An obstruction of the intestines causing immobility of the intestines.

Intravenous – Pertaining to the inside of a vein.

IV – Abbreviation for the term intravenous.

Jejunum – The middle ten feet of small intestine extending from the duodenum to the ileum; the part responsible for digestion.

Keratin – A fibrous sulfur containing protein that is the primary component of the skin, hair, nails, and enamel of the teeth.

Kilogram – Measure of weight equal to 2.2 pounds.

Lactose intolerant – A sensitivity disorder resulting in the inability to digest lactose (milk sugar) from dairy products because of inadequate production of, or defect in the enzyme lactase.

Lap-Band® – Brand name for a particular adjustable gastric band.

Laparoscopy – Method of visualizing and treating intra-abdominal problems with long fiber-optic instruments.

Large intestine – Lower portion of the intestinal tract. In the large intestine, excess fluids are absorbed and a firm stool is formed. The colon may absorb protein, when necessary.

LDL cholesterol – Abbreviation for low-density lipoprotein. LDL is a plasma protein provided by the liver, and delivers lipids and cholesterol to the body tissues.

Magnesium – A silver white mineral element.

Metabolism – The aggregate of all chemical processes that take place in living organisms resulting in growth, generation of energy, elimination of wastes, and other body functions as they relate to the distribution of nutrients in the blood after digestion.

Morbid Obesity – Body Mass Index of 40 or more, which is roughly equivalent to 100 pounds or more over ideal body weight.

Morbid – Pertaining to disease, illness, increased risk of death.

Mortality – Pertaining to death.

Multi-disciplinary approach – Team approach to evaluation and treatment of clinically severe obesity; includes surgical, internal medicine, nutrition, behavioral, and exercise physiology assessment and treatment.

Myocardial infarction (MI) – necrosis (dead tissue) of a portion of a cardiac muscle caused by an obstruction in a coronary artery through narrowing of the artery, a blood clot, or a spasm. Also called heart attack.

Nasogastric tube – Any tube passed into the stomach through the nose.

Negative conditioning – A form of behavior modification in which the presentment of something immediately after occurrence of a particular behavior, will decrease the rate of recurrence of the behavior.

NIH – National Institutes of Health.

NIH Consensus Report – Summaries of meetings regarding clinically severe obesity and the assessment and treatment of obesity; issued periodically by NIH.

Nitrosamines – Potentially cancer causing compounds produced by reactions of nitrites with amines or amides normally present in the body.

NSAID – Non-steroidal anti-inflammatory drug.

OB specialist – A physician who specializes in obstetrics (the care of pregnant women).

Obesity – Pertaining to excessive weight or adipose tissue.

Obstruction – Narrowing of an anastomosis or segment of gastrointestinal tract which slows normal passage of food or waste materials.

Obstructive sleep apnea – A sleep disorder characterized by periods in which breathing is absent. The person is monetarily unable to contract respiratory muscles or to maintain airflow through the nose or mouth, and may experience recurrent sleep interruptions, choking and gasping spells on awakening, and drowsiness caused by loss of normal sleep. The physical obstruction contributing to this disorder is usually in the upper airways, and is generally a result of obesity.

Osteoarthritis – A form of arthritis in which one or many joints undergo degenerative changes. Arthritis is an inflammatory condition of the joints characterized by pain, swelling, heat, redness, and limitation of movement.

Panniculus – a sheet or layer of tissue: the superficial fascia which contains an abundance of fat deposit in its areolar substance.

Panic attack – An episode of acute anxiety that occurs unpredictably with feelings of intense apprehension or terror, accompanied by dizziness, sweating, trembling, and chest pain or palpitations. The attack may last several minutes and may occur again in certain situations.

Peristalsis – The coordinated, rhythmic serial contraction of smooth muscle that forces food through the digestive tract, bile through the bile duct, and urine through the ureters.

PCA – Patient controlled analgesia. A drug delivery system that dispenses a preset intravascular dose of a narcotic pain medication when the patient pushes a switch on an electric cord. The patient administers a dose of narcotic when the need for pain relief arises. A lockout interval automatically inactivates the system if the patient tries to increase the amount of narcotic within the preset period.

pH level – Abbreviation for potential hydrogen, a scale representative of the relative acidity (or alkilinity) of a solution, in which a value of 7.0 is neutral, below 7.0 is acid, and above 7.0 is alkaline.

Plastic surgery – The alteration, replacement, or restoration of visible parts of the body, performed to correct a structural or cosmetic defect. The medical term "plastic" refers to something that is conformable, or capable of being molded.

Pneumonia – An acute inflammation of the lungs, often caused by inhaled bacteria, viruses, or fungi.

Polycystic ovary syndrome – An endocrine disturbance characterized by lack of ovulation, lack of menstruation, excessive body or facial hair, and infertility.

Post-traumatic stress disorder (PTSD) – A disorder characterized by an acute emotional response to a traumatic event or situation involving severe environmental stress, such as a natural disaster, airplane crash, serious automobile accident, military combat, or physical torture.

Potassium – An alkali metal element. Helps to regulate neuromuscular excitability and muscle contraction.

Psychotherapy – Evaluation and treatment of mentally related disorders.

Pulmonary – Pertaining to the lungs.

Pulmonary embolism (PE) – The blockage of a pulmonary artery by fat, air, tumor tissue, or blood clot that usually arises from a peripheral vein (most frequently one of the deep veins of the legs).

Pulse-oximetry monitor – A device that measures the amount of saturated hemoglobin in the tissue capillaries.

Pylorus – The pylorus is a small round muscle located at the outlet of the stomach and the entrance to the duodenum (the first section of the small intestine). It closes the stomach outlet while food is being digested into a smaller, more easily absorbed form. When food is properly digested, the pylorus opens and allows the contents of the stomach into the duodenum.

Rapid gastric emptying – See Dumping Syndrome.

Respiratory dysfunction – Pertains to a lung or lungs that are unable to function normally.

Roux-en-Y gastric bypass – A surgical method of reconnecting the stomach and upper small intestines in roughly a Y shape.

Saline solution – A solution containing sodium chloride.

Sclerotherapy – The use of sclerosing (tissue hardening) chemicals to treat conditions such as hemorrhoids, or esophageal ulcers.

Sedation – An induced state of quiet, calmness, or sleep, as by means of a sedative or hypnotic medication.

Small intestine – The small intestine is about 15 to 20 feet long (4.5 to 6 meters) and is where the majority of the absorption of the nutrients from food takes place. The small intestine is made up of three sections: the duodenum, the jejunum, and the ileum.

Spasm – Twitching or involuntary contraction of a specified sort.

Staples – Surgically sterile devices for connecting tissue; usually permanent and made of stainless steel or titanium.

Stenosis – An abnormal condition characterized by the constriction or narrowing of an opening or passageway in a body structure.

Stomach – The stomach, situated at the top of the abdomen, normally holds just over 3 pints (about 1500 ml) of food from a single meal. Here the food is mixed with an acid that is produced to assist in digestion. In the stomach, acid and other digestive juices are added to the ingested food to facilitate breakdown of complex proteins, fats, and carbohydrates into small, more absorbable units.

Stress urinary incontinence – The state in which an individual experiences a loss of urine of less than 50 ml occurring with increased abdominal pressure, such as experienced during coughing, sneezing, laughing, and lifting.

Stricture – Narrowing of anastomosis or section of intestine; often related to inflammation, external pressure, or scarring.

Stroke – Also known as cerebrovascualar accident (CVA). An abnormal condition of the brain characterized by bleeding in the brain that may permanently damage tissue resulting in a variety of deficits.

Therapy – Treatment.

Thrush – Candidiasis of the tissues of the mouth characterized by the appearance of creamy white patches of mucus on an inflamed tongue or gums.

TPN (total parenteral nutrition) – The administration of a nutritionally adequate hypertonic solution through an indwelling catheter. The procedure is used in situations including prolonged coma, severe uncontrolled malabsorption, extensive burns, and other condition in which feeding by mouth cannot provide adequate amounts of nutrition.

Type II diabetes – Also known as Type II Diabetes Mellitus. A disorder of glucose and insulin metabolism in which patients are not insulin dependent, although they may use insulin for correction of symptomatic hyperglycemia (high blood sugar). Approximately 60%-90% of these patients are obese, and the condition is often improved by weight loss.

Ultrasound – Sound waves at the very high frequency over 20 kHz (vibrations per second).

Valve – A valve at the entrance to the stomach from the esophagus allows the food to enter while keeping the acid-laden food from "refluxing" back into the esophagus, causing damage and pain. Another valve separates the small and large intestines to keep bacteria-laden colon contents from coming back into the small intestine.

For additional definitions and explanations, please visit our website at:

www.littlevictoriespress.com
and click on "extended glossary."

Chapter Eighteen

➤ REFERENCE CITATIONS ➤

Chapter Two – Enlightenment

1. Staple line buttressing material developed by R. Baker, J. Foote and Gore and Associates, Seamguard®.

2. Baker, R., Foote, J., Kemmeter, P., Brady, R., Vroegop, T., Serveld, M. (2004). The science of stapling and leaks. *Obesity Surgery,* 14(10). 1290-8.

Chapter Three – The New and Improved, Amazing, All Natural Lemon Diet

1. Sturm, R., Ringel, J., Andreyeva, T. (2004). Increasing obesity rates and disability trends. *Health Affairs,* 23 (2). 199-205; United States. Centers for Disease Control, National Center for Health Statistics. Overweight prevalence. (2002). Washington DC: US Government Printing Office; Buchwald, H., Avidor, Y., Braunwald, E., et al. (2004). Bariatric surgery: a systematic review and meta-analysis. *Journal of the American Medical Association,* 292(14). 1724-37; Liping, L., Meydani, M. (2003). Angiogenesis inhibitors may regulate adiposity. *Nutrition Reviews,* 61(11). 384-387; Rosner, S. (2002). Obesity: the disease of the twenty-first century. *International Journal of Obesity Related Metabolic Disorders,* 26. S2-S4; http://www.ASBS.org/html/rationale/ rationale.html (Rationale for the Surgical Treatment of Obesity).

2. http://www.familystudies.org/alcoholism&genetics.htm (a site of the University of California — San Francisco, Department of Neurology, Gallo Clinic and Research Center – Human Genetics Project); Shuckit, M. (1999). New findings on the genetics of alcoholism. *Journal of the American Medical Association,* 281 (20). 1875-1876; Bouchard, C. (1994). The Genetics of Obesity. Boca Raton: CRC Press. 245.

3. United States. Alcohol Alert: National Institute on Alcohol Abuse and Alcoholism. (1992). No. 18, PH 357. Washington DC: U.S. Government Printing Office.

4. Cardon, L., Carmelli, D., Fabsitz, R., Reed, T. (1994). Genetic and environmental correlations between obesity and body fat distribution in adult male twins. *Human Biology,* 663. 465-479.

5. Jensen, G., Rogers, J. (1998). Obesity in older persons. *American Dietetic Association Journal,* (98). 1308-131.

6. United States. Surgeon General's call to action to prevent and decrease overweight and obesity. (2001). Washington DC: U.S. Government Printing Office.

7. Schwartz, M., Chambliss, H., Brownell, K, Blair, S., Billington, C. (2003). Weight bias among health professionals specializing in obesity. *Obesity Research,* 11. 1033-1039; Teachman, B., Brownell, K. (2001). Implicit anti-fat bias among health professionals: is anyone immune? *International Journal of Obesity Related Metabolic Disorders,* 25. 1525-1531; Loomis, G., Connolly, K., Clinch, C., Djuric, D. (2001) Attitudes and practices of military family physicians regarding obesity. *Military Medicine,* 166. 121-125.

8. Puhl, R., Brownell, K. (2001). Bias, Discrimination, and Obesity. *Obesity Research,* 9(12). 788-805.

9. Garner, D., Wooley, S. (1991). Confronting the failure of behavioral and dietary treatments for obesity. *Clinical Psychology Review,* 11(6). 729-780.

10. http://www.med.umich.edu/opm/newspage/2003/yoyodiet.htm. (Study links yo-yo dieting to poor post-menopause heart health.)

11. http://www.nih.gov/nihrecord/01_18_2005/story09.htm (Ghosh, A. (2205). Focus on women: seminar explores obesity research, stigma).

12. Perri, M., Fuller, P. (1995). Success and failure in the treatment of obesity: where do we go from here? *Med Exerc Nutr Health,* 4. 255-272; National Task Force on the Prevention and Treatment of Obesity: very low calorie diets. *(1993). Journal of the American Medical Association,* 270. 967-974; Safer, D. (1991). Diet, behavior modification and exercise: a review of obesity treatments from a long term perspective. *South Med J,* 84(12). 1470-4; Weintraub, M., et al. (1992). Long-term weight control study IV (weeks 156-190): The second double-blind phase. *Clin Pharmacol Ther,* 51. 608-614; Powers, P., Dietel, M. ed. (1989). Conservative treatments for morbid obesity, in surgery for the morbidly obese patient. Lea & Feibiger: Philadelphia. 27-37; United States. National Institutes of Health. Clinical guidelines on the identification, evaluation, and treatment of overweight and obesity in adults: The evidence report. (1998). Bethesda, MD: US Department of Health and Human Services; Jain, A. (2004). What works for obesity? A summary of the research behind obesity interventions. BMJ Publishing Group: London, England.

13. *Id.*

14. . Hell, E., Miller, K., Moorehead, M., et al. (2000). Evaluation of health status and quality of life after bariatric surgery: comparison of standard roux-en-y gastric bypass, vertical banded gastroplasty, and laparoscopic adjustable silicone gastric banding. *Obesity Surgery,* 10. 214-19; United States. National Institutes of Health. Consensus Statement 84. Bethesda, MD: US Department of Health and Human Services.

15. Finkelstein, E., Fiebelkorn, I., Wang, G. (2004). State-level estimates of annual medical expenditures attributable to obesity. *Obesity Research,* Jan. 18-24; Craig, B., Tseng, D. (2002). The cost-effectiveness of bariatric surgery. *American Journal of Internal Medicine, 113.* 491-8; Allison, D., Zannolli, R., Vienkat, K. (1999). The direct healthcare costs of obesity in the United States. *American Journal of Public Health,* 89. 1194-1199.

16. Lakdawalla, D., Bhattacharya, J., Dana, P. (2004). Are the young becoming more disabled? *Health Affairs,* 23. 168-176; Sturm, R., Ringel, J., Andreyeva, T. (2004). Increasing obesity rates and disability trends. *Health Affairs,* 23(2) 199-205.

17. Weber, M., Muller, M., Bucher, T., et al. (2004). Laparoscopic gastric bypass is superior to laparoscopic gastric banding for treatment of morbid obesity. *Annals of Surgery,* 240(6). 975-983; Hell, E., Miller, K., Moorehead, M., et al. (2000). Evaluation of health status and quality of life after bariatric surgery: comparison of standard roux-en-y gastric bypass, vertical banded gastroplasty, and laparoscopic adjustable silicone gastric banding. *Obesity Surgery,* 10. 214-19; Pories, W., Swanson, M., MacDonald, K., et al. (1995). Who would have thought it? An operation proves to be the most effective therapy for adult onset diabetes mellitus. *Annals of Surgery,* 222(3). 339-50; Chapman, A., Kiroff, G., Game, P., et al. (2004). Laparoscopic adjustable gastric banding in the treatment of obesity: a systematic literature review. *Surgery,* 135(3). 326-51.

18. Chapman, A., Kiroff, G., Game, P., et al. (2004). Laparoscopic adjustable gastric banding in the treatment of obesity: a systematic literature review. *Surgery,*135(3). 326-51.

19. Sapala, J., Wood, M., Schuhknecht, M., Sapala, M. (2003). Fatal pulmonary embolism after bariatric operations for morbid obesity: a 24-year retrospective analysis. *Obesity Surgery,* 13(6). 819-25.

20. Luukkonen, P., Kalima, T., Kivilaakso, F.. (1990). Decreased risk of gastric stump carcinoma after partial gastrectomy supplemented with bile diversion. *Hepatogastroenterology*, 37(4). 392-394; Lacaine, F., Houry, S., Huguier, M. (1992). Stomach cancer after partial gastrectomy for benign ulcer disease: a critical analysis of epidemiological reports. *Hepatogastroenterology*, 39(1). 4-8; Tersmette, A., Giardiello, F., Tytgat, G., Offerhaus, G. (1995). Carcinogenesis after remote peptic ulcer surgery: the long-term prognosis of partial gastrectomy. *Scandinavian Journal of Gastroenterology Supplement*, 212. 96-99.

21. Chapman, A., Kiroff, G., Game, P., et al. (2004). Laparoscopic adjustable gastric banding in the treatment of obesity: a systematic literature review. *Surgery*,135(3). 326-51.

22. Tanenberg, R., Pories, W. (2002). Surgery for obesity. *Diabetes Forecast*, 55(4). 81-86; Chapman, A., Kiroff, G., Game, P., et al. (2004). Laparoscopic adjustable gastric banding in the treatment of obesity: a systematic literature review. *Surgery*,135(3). 326-51; Sapala, J., Wood, M., Schuhknecht, M., Sapala, M. (2003). Fatal pulmonary embolism after bariatric operations for morbid obesity: a 24-year retrospective analysis. *Obesity Surgery*, 13(6). 819-25; Melinek, J., Livingston, E., Cortina, G., Fishbein, M. (2002). Autopsy findings following gastric bypass surgery for morbid obesity. *Archives of Pathology & Laboratory Medicine*, 126(9). 1091-5; http://www.memorial-health.net – (Possible complications from gastric bypass surgery.); Spaw, A., Husted, J. (2005). Bleeding after laparoscopic gastric bypass: case report and literature review. *Surgery for Obesity and Related Diseases*, 1(2). 99-103;

23. Ritter, M., Harty, L., Davis, K., Meding, J., Berend, M. (2003). Simultaneous bilateral, staged bilateral, and unilateral total knee arthroplasty: a survival analysis. *Journal of Bone and Joint Surgery*, 85-A(8). 1532-7; Sheppeard, H., Cleak, D., Ward, D., O'Connor, B. (1980). A review of mortality and morbidity in elderly patients following Charnley total hip replacement. *Archives of Orthopaedic and Traumatic Surgery*, 97(4). 243-8; Chapman, A., Kiroff, G., Game, P., et al. (2004). Laparoscopic adjustable gastric banding in the treatment of obesity: a systematic literature review. *Surgery*,135(3). 326-51.

24. Flum, D., Dellinger, E. (2004). Impact of gastric bypass operation on survival: a population based analysis. *Journal American College of Surgery*, 199. 543-551; http://www.njbariatricspc.com/tips/risk.asp.

25. Buchwald, H., Avidor, Y., Braunwald, E., et al. (2004). Bariatric surgery: a systematic review and meta-analysis. *Journal of the American Medical Association*, 292(14). 1724-37.

26. Buchwald, H., Avidor, Y., Braunwald, E., et al. (2004). Bariatric surgery: a systematic review and meta-analysis. *Journal of the American Medical Association*, 292(14). 1724-37.

27. Pories, W., Swanson, M., MacDonald, K., et al. (1995). Who would have thought it? An operation proves to be the most effective therapy for adult onset diabetes mellitus. *Annals of Surgery*, 222(3). 339-50.

28. Spivak, H., Hewitt, M., Onn, A., Half, E. (2005). Weight loss and improvement of obesity-related illness in 500 U.S. patients following laparoscopic adjustable gastric banding procedure. *American Journal of Surgery*, 189(1). 27-32; Frigg, A., Peterli, R., Peters, T., Ackermann, C., Tondelli, P. (2004). Reduction in co-morbidities 4 years after laparoscopic adjustable gastric banding. *Obesity Surgery*, 14(2). 216-23.

29. Chapman, A., Kiroff, G., Game, P., et al. (2004). Laparoscopic adjustable gastric banding in the treatment of obesity: a systematic literature review. *Surgery*,135(3). 326-51.

30. http://www.asbs.org/html/story/chapter3.html

31. Hall, J., Watts, J., O'Brien, P., et al. (1990). Gastric surgery for morbid obesity. Adelaide Study. *Annals of Surgery*, 211. 419-27.

32. Perri, M., Fuller, P. (1995). Success and failure in the treatment of obesity: where do we go from here? *Med Exerc Nutr Health*, 4. 255-272; National Task Force on the Prevention and Treatment of Obesity: very low calorie diets. *(1993). Journal of the American Medical Association*, 270. 967-974; Safer, D. (1991). Diet, behavior modification and exercise. A review of obesity treatments from a long term perspective. *South Med J*, 84(12). 1470-4; Weintraub, M., et al. (1992). Long-term weight control study IV (weeks 156-190) The second double-blind phase. *Clin Pharmacol Ther*, 51. 608-614; Powers, P., Dietel, M. ed. (1989). Conservative treatments for morbid obesity, in surgery for the morbidly obese patient. Lea & Feibiger: Philadelphia. 27-37; United States. National Institutes of Health. Clinical guidelines on the identification, evaluation, and treatment of overweight and obesity in adults: The evidence report. (1998). Bethesda, MD: US Department of Health and Human Services; Jain, A. (2004). What works for obesity? A summary of the research behind obesity interventions. BMJ

Publishing Group: London, England; Pories, W., Swanson, M., MacDonald, K., et al. (1995). Who would have thought it? An operation proves to be the most effective therapy for adult onset diabetes mellitus. *Annals of Surgery*, 222(3). 339-50.

33. Pories, W., Swanson, M., MacDonald, K., et al. (1995). Who would have thought it? An operation proves to be the most effective therapy for adult onset diabetes mellitus. *Annals of Surgery*, 222(3). 339-50.

34. Pories, W., Swanson, M., MacDonald, K., et al. (1995). Who would have thought it? An operation proves to be the most effective therapy for adult onset diabetes mellitus. *Annals of Surgery*, 222(3). 339-50; Barakat, H., McLendon, V., Marks, R., Pories, W., Heath, J., Carpenter, J. (1992). Influence of morbid obesity on non-insulin-dependent diabetes mellitus on high-density lipoprotein composition and subpopulation distribution. *Metabolism,* 41(1). 37-41.

35. http://www.ASBS.org/html/rationale/rationale.html (Rationale for the Surgical Treatment of Morbid Obesity).

Chapter Five – Auto Eject

1. http://www.mayoclinic.com.

2. *Mosby's Medical, Nursing & Allied Health Dictionary*, (6th ed.). (2002). St. Louis: Mosby.

3. http://www.healthlink.mcw.edu.

4. http://www.healthlink.mcw.edu

Chapter Nine – Separation Anxiety

1. Charles Horton Cooley (1864-1929). Cooley, C.H. (1902). *Human Nature and the Social Order.* New York: Scribner's; Henslen, J.M. (2005). *Sociology: A Down-to-Earth Approach.* (7th ed.). Boston: Pearson Allyn and Bacon; Best, S. (2003). *A Beginners Guide to Social Theory.* Thousand Oaks: Sage Publications.

2. *Id.*

3. Erving Goffman (1922-1982). Goffman, E. (1959). *The Presentation of Self in Everyday Life.* New York: Doubleday; Henslen, J.M. (2005). *Sociology: A Down-to-Earth Approach.* (7th ed.). Boston: Pearson Allyn and Bacon; Best, S. (2003). *A Beginners Guide to Social Theory.* Thousand Oaks: Sage Publications.

4. *See* Glossary for definition. Henslen, J.M. (2005). *Sociology: A Down-to-Earth Approach.* (7th ed.). Boston: Pearson Allyn and Bacon.

Chapter Fourteen – Shrink! Shrank! Shrunk!!

1. http://www.ASBS.org

2. http://www.ASPS.org

3. http://www.ASAPS.org

4. http://www.ASPS.org

Chapter Fifteen – The Final Battle: Defeat of the Clones

1. Eisenstein, J., Greenberg, A. (2003). Ghrelin: update 2003. *Nutrition Reviews,* 61(3). 101-104; Tassone, F., Broglio, F., Destefanis, S., Rovere, S., et al. (2003). Neuroendocrine and metabolic effects of acute ghrelin administration in human obesity. *Journal of Clinical Endocrinology and Metabolism,* 88(11). 5478-83; Tschop, M., Statnick, M., Suter, T., Heiman, M. (2002). GH-releasing peptide-2 increases fat mass in mice lacking NPY: indication for a crucial mediating role of hypothalamic agouti-related protein. *Endocrinology,* 143. 555-568.

2. Cummings, D., Weigle, D., Frayo, R., et al. (2002). Plasma ghrelin levels after diet-induced weight loss or gastric bypass surgery. *New England Journal of Medicine,* 346. 1623-1630; Eisenstein, J., Greenberg, A. (2003). Ghrelin: update 2003. *Nutrition Reviews,* 61(3). 101-104; Hanusch-Enserer, U., Cauza, E., Brabant, G., Dunky, A., et al. (2004). Plasma ghrelin in obesity before and after weight loss after laparascopical adjustable gastric banding. *Journal of Clinical Endocrinology and Metabolism,* 89(7). 3352-8.

3. Carlini, V., Manzon, M., Varas, M., Cragnolini, A., et al. (2002). Ghrelin increases anxiety-like behavior and memory retention in rats. *Biochemical and Biophysical Research Communications,* 299(5). 739-43.

4. Arner, P. (2000). Obesity – a genetic disease of adipose tissue? *British Journal of Nutrition,* 83(1). S9-16; Bouchard, C. (1993). Genes and body fat. *American Journal of Human Biology,* 5. 425-432.

Chapter Seventeen – Glossary

Mosby's Medical, Nursing & Allied Health Dictionary, (6th ed.). (2002). St. Louis: Mosby.

Stedman's Medical Dictionary, (26th ed.). (1995). Baltimore: Williams & Wilkins.

Taber's Cyclopedic Medical Dictionary, (17th ed.). (1993). Philadelphia: F.A. Davis Company.

They can conquer who believe they can.

VIRGIL

Quick Order Form

THE *Real*
SKINNY ON WEIGHT LOSS SURGERY

An Indispensable Guide to What You Can REALLY Expect!

Fax orders: 517-589-5535

Postal orders: **Little Victories Press, 4371 Kinneville Road, Suite 200, Onondaga, Michigan 49264.**

Email orders: **orders@www.LittleVictoriesPress.com**

Visit us at our web site: **www.LittleVictoriesPress.com**

Please send me more FREE information on:

☐ Upcoming books from LVP   ☐ Speaking engagements   ☐ Consulting

Name: _____

Address: _____

City/State/Zip: _____

Telephone: _____

Email Address: _____

Please send me _____ copies of this book at $19.95 each for myself or to share with others!

Physicians' offices: Please contact us for special rates

Sales Tax: Please add 6% Michigan Sales Tax to your total order

Shipping by Air:
US: $4.00 for the first book, and $2.00 for each additional product shipped at the same time.

International: $9.00 for the first book, and $5.00 for each additional product shipped at the same time.

Payment: I have enclosed a check or money order in the amount of $_____ made payable to Little Victories Press.
For credit card orders, please see web site, or call us directly. 1-866-LVBOOK4 (1-866-582-6654).

On those days when you think this is hard...

remember... it's supposed to be,

or everyone would be doing it...

that's what makes it so great.

ANONYMOUS